O A R L
OXFORD AMERICAN RHEUMATOLOGY LIBRARY

Ankylosing Spondylitis

OARL
OXFORD AMERICAN RHEUMATOLOGY LIBRARY

Ankylosing Spondylitis

Muhammad Asim Khan, MD, MACP, FRCP

Professor of Medicine
Case Western Reserve University
Cleveland, OH

MetroHealth Medical Center
Department of Medicine, Division of Rheumatology
Cleveland, OH

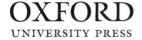

OXFORD
UNIVERSITY PRESS

OXFORD
UNIVERSITY PRESS

Oxford University Press, Inc., publishes works that further
Oxford University's objective of excellence
in research, scholarship, and education.

Oxford New York

Auckland Cape Town Dar es Salaam Hong Kong Karachi
Kuala Lumpur Madrid Melbourne Mexico City Nairobi
New Delhi Shanghai Taipei Toronto

With offices in
Argentina Austria Brazil Chile Czech Republic France Greece
Guatemala Hungary Italy Japan Poland Portugal Singapore
South Korea Switzerland Thailand Turkey Ukraine Vietnam

Copyright © 2009 by Muhammad Asim Khan
All Rights Reserved

Published by Oxford University Press, Inc.
198 Madison Avenue, New York, New York 10016
www.oup.com

Oxford is a registered trademark of Oxford University Press

Library of Congress Cataloging-in-Publication Data

Khan, Muhammad Asim.
Ankylosing spondylitis / Muhammad Asim Khan.
p. ; cm.—(Oxford American rheumatology library)
Includes bibliographical references and index.
ISBN 978-0-19-536807-9

1. Ankylosing spondylitis.   I. Title. II. Series.
[DNLM: 1. Spondylitis, Ankylosing—diagnosis. 2. Spondylitis, Ankylosing—therapy.
3. Early Diagnosis. WE 725 K450 2008]
RD771.A5K49 2008
616.7'3—dc22   2008027171

9 8 7 6 5 4 3 2 1
Printed in the United States of America
on acid-free paper

Dedication

I dedicate this book to the fond memories of my father
M. S. Umar Khan
1914–2008

Preface

This book on ankylosing spondylitis (or AS for short), as a part of the new *Oxford American Rheumatology Library* series, provides practical, evidence-based information for health-care professionals. AS is the archetype and the most serious and common form of a group of inflammatory diseases called spondyloarthropathies (SpA) that as a group are almost as common as rheumatoid arthritis. The presenting clinical manifestations of SpA are very wide and heterogeneous, so patients with these conditions are being seen by health-care professionals ranging from primary care physicians to medical and surgical specialists.

The current mean delay in the diagnosis of AS varies between 5 and 10 years and is often longer in women. The book describes clinical manifestations, with an emphasis on clinical pointers for early diagnosis, which are sorely needed with the recent availability of effective treatment. It is designed to be a helpful companion for the health-care professionals to whom most patients with AS present, often repeatedly before an accurate diagnosis is made and appropriate treatment is initiated. It provides comprehensive coverage of current treatment options, including the latest biologic therapies.

I hope that health-care providers will find the information provided in this book to be clinically useful in helping them make an early diagnosis of AS and related SpA and provide appropriate management. I have also written a companion book on AS for educating patients and their families about this disease (*Ankylosing Spondylitis: The Facts*, Oxford University Press, 2002).

I may add that I myself have suffered from AS for more than 52 years, and my main academic research interest has dealt with AS and related SpA during my 43 years as a physician. I have also relied on many of my earlier publications in writing this book, and some of those publications are listed at the end.

I am grateful to Dr. Irving Kushner and to many international colleagues (too many to list here) for collaborative efforts during the past four decades, most recently to Dr. Mazen Elyan.

Contents

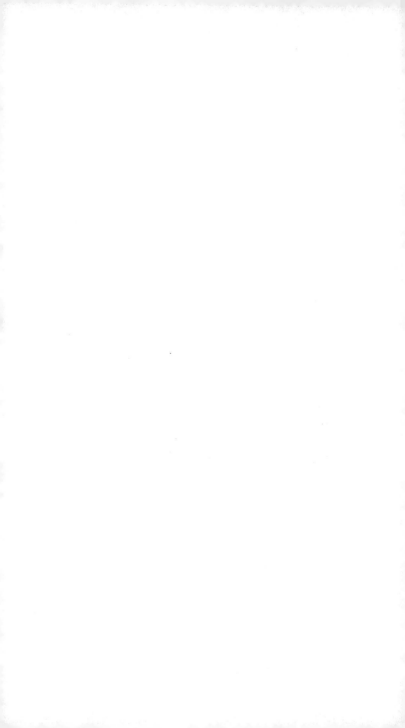

List of Abbreviations

ACR20	American College of Rheumatology ≥20% Response Criteria
ADL	activities of daily living
AS	ankylosing spondylitis
ASAS	Assessment in Ankylosing Spondylitis International Working Group
ASAS20	≥20% ASAS Response Criteria
ASIF	AS International Federation
BASDAI	Bath Ankylosing Spondylitis Disease Activity Index
BASFI	Bath Ankylosing Spondylitis Functional Index
BASMI	Bath Ankylosing Spondylitis Metrology Index
CD	Crohn's disease
COX	cyclooxygenase
CRP	C-reactive protein
CT	computed tomography
DCARD	disease-controlling antirheumatic drug
DCART	disease-controlling antirheumatic therapy
DEXA	dual energy x-ray absorptiometry
DIP	distal interphalangeal joints
DISH	diffuse idiopathic skeletal hyperostosis
DMARD	disease-modifying antirheumatic drug
DMART	disease-modifying antirheumatic therapy
EMEA	European Medicines Agency (European equivalent of FDA)
ERA	enthesitis-related arthritis
ESR	erythrocyte sedimentation rate
ESSG	European Spondyloarthropathy Study Group
FACIT	Functional Assessment of Chronic Illness Therapy
FDA	U.S. Food and Drug Administration
GRAPPA	Group for Research and Treatment of Psoriasis and Psoriatic Arthritis
HAQ	Health Assessments Questionnaire
HAQ-S	spondylitis-specific HAQ measure
HLA-B27	human leukocyte antigen B27
IBD	chronic inflammatory bowel disease
IBP	inflammatory back pain

ICER	incremental cost-effectiveness ratio
IL23R	interleukin-23 receptor
INH	isoniazid
JIA	juvenile idiopathic arthritis
LR	likelihood ratio
MFI	Multidimensional Fatigue Inventory
MHC	major histocompatibility complex
MOMP	major outer membrane protein
MRI	magnetic resonance imaging
mSASSS	Modified Stoke Ankylosing Spondylitis Spine Score
MTX	methotrexate
NICE	National Institute for Health and Clinical Excellence (UK)
NIH	National Institutes of Health (U.S.)
NSAIDs	nonsteroidal anti-inflammatory drugs
OA	osteoarthritis
OASIS	Outcome Assessments in Ankylosing Spondylitis International Study
PASS	patient acceptable symptom state
PCR	polymerase chain reaction
POEMS	polyneuropathy, organomegaly, endocrinopathy, monoclonal gammopathy, and skin changes syndrome
PPD	purified protein derivative
PsA	psoriatic arthritis
PT	physical therapy
QALY	quality-adjusted life-year
QOL	quality of life
RA	rheumatoid arthritis
ReA	reactive arthritis
SAA	Spondylitis Association of America
SAPHO	synovitis acne pustulosis hyperostosis osteitis syndrome
SEA	seronegative enthesitis and arthritis syndrome
SI joint	sacroiliac joint
SMARD	symptom-modifying antirheumatic drug
SMART	symptom-modifying antirheumatic therapy
SpA	spondyloarthropathies (spondyloarthritis)
SPARC	Spondyloarthritis Research Consortium of Canada
SPARTAN	Spondyloarthritis Research and Treatment Network
STIR	short tau inversion recovery
TB	tuberculosis
TNF-α	tumor necrosis factor-α

Chapter 1

Introductory overview: Ankylosing spondylitis

Ankylosing spondylitis (AS) is a chronic systemic inflammatory disease that shows a predilection for involvement of the axial skeleton: the sacroiliac joints, vertebral column, chest wall, and hip and shoulder girdles (Fig. 1.1).[1-3] Its name is derived from the Greek *angkylos*, meaning "bent" (but now it has come to imply fusion), and *spondylos*, meaning "spinal vertebrae." It is the predominant member or prototype and often the main outcome of a family of related diseases termed the spondyloarthropathies (SpA), a group of overlapping inflammatory rheumatologic diseases that show a tendency for inflammation of the axial skeleton, entheses (bony insertions of ligaments and tendons; singular is enthesis), and peripheral joints.[4,5] They may also involve extraskeletal structures such as the eyes, skin, gut, and genitourinary tract.

The pathogenesis of AS is poorly understood, but it is multifactorial, with a strong genetic predisposition that is associated with HLA-B27; approximately three-fourths of the total genetic risk of developing AS has been determined.[6-8] Among the possible environmental triggers, infections have long been suspected, but no association has yet been established. The close relationships of AS with psoriasis and Crohn's disease (both clinical as well as subclinical or asymptomatic forms) imply potential involvement of an immune reaction in the gut and/or skin that may be influenced by microbial reactions in genetically susceptible individuals to result in AS.

The inflammation usually starts in the sacroiliac joints, lasting a few days to many weeks. Initially it may fluctuate from one side to the other, causing what the patient may describe as "alternating buttock pain," before it extends to involve the spine. Chronic back pain and progressive stiffening of the spine are usually the first symptoms that lead the patient to seek medical help (Table 1.1). These symptoms usually begin insidiously in late adolescence and early adulthood, worsen with physical inactivity or prolonged rest, and are generally eased with exercise or a hot shower.

Detection of sacroiliac joint involvement (sacroiliitis) on musculoskeletal imaging (conventional radiography [Fig. 1.2], magnetic resonance imaging, or computed tomography) in the presence of clinical manifestations is virtually diagnostic for AS.[9] There is often associated inflammation (enthesitis) of discovertebral, apophyseal, costovertebral, and costotransverse joints and the paravertebral ligamentous structures, usually resulting in gradual but progressive limitation of spinal mobility and chest expansion.

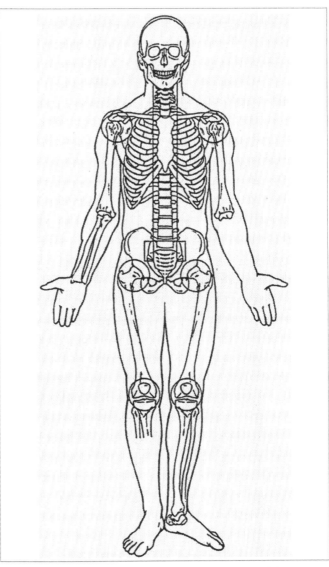

Figure 1.1 This drawing indicates the sites that may be involved in ankylosing spondylitis. The most commonly involved sites are the sacroiliac joints and the spine (marked by rectangles). Less commonly involved sites are the hip and shoulder joints, and still less often the knee joints (marked by circles). Reprinted with permission from Khan MA. *Ankylosing Spondylitis: The Facts*. Oxford: Oxford University Press; 2002.

Peripheral joints are less often involved, although large joints such as the hips and shoulders are affected in about one-third of patients. Some patients may also show extra-articular manifestations, most commonly one or more episodes of acute anterior uveitis.

A variety of clinical presentations, such as enthesitis, peripheral arthritis, or acute anterior uveitis, may antedate back symptoms in some patients. Enthesitis may cause pain and tenderness over the anterior chest wall, spinal processes, iliac crests, and sites of bony insertions of the Achilles and patellar tendons and plantar fascia. Early AS should be strongly suspected when a person, often young, presents with inflammatory back pain plus at least a couple of other typical features of SpA, such as acute anterior uveitis and enthesitis.

Table 1.1 Clinical features of ankylosing spondylitis

- Chronic inflammatory back pain and stiffness of insidious onset in late adolescence and early adulthood; these symptoms worsen with prolonged rest or physical inactivity but are eased on physical activity
- Generally good symptomatic response to anti-inflammatory dose of NSAIDs and regular physical exercise
- Tendency for inflammation at sites of bony insertions for tendons and ligaments (enthesitis), with adjacent subchondral bone edema (osteitis) and adjacent synovitis
- Characteristic radiographic sacroiliitis and variable progression to spondylitis
- Gradually progressive limitation of spinal mobility and later even chest expansion
- Increased risk of anterior ocular inflammation (acute anterior uveitis)
- Increased familial incidence
- Strong association with HLA-B27, but strength of this association varies appreciably among various racial and ethnic groups
- No association with rheumatoid factor and antinuclear antibodies
- Sometimes association with psoriasis, ulcerative colitis, Crohn's disease, and reactive arthritis
- Occasional extraskeletal manifestations include aortitis, heart block, apical pulmonary fibrosis, or cauda equina syndrome

(a)   (b)

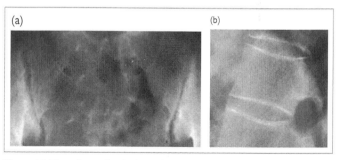

Figure 1.2 These figures show radiographic evidence of involvement of the sacroiliac joints and spine in ankylosing spondylitis and related spondyloarthropathies. (A) This pelvic radiograph shows evidence of bilateral sacroiliitis with fuzziness and erosions of joint margins and adjacent bony sclerosis; these changes are more prominent on the iliac side of the joint. (B) This radiograph of the lumbar spine (lateral view) shows squaring of the anterior corners of the vertebral bodies and a faint image of possible early changes that will result in syndesmophyte formation.

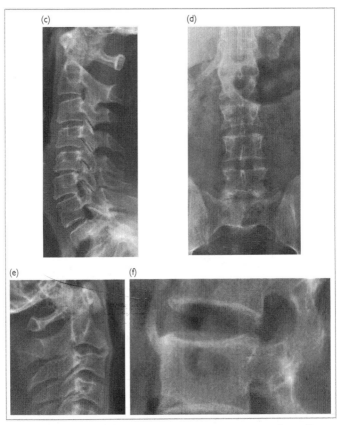

Figure 1.2 (C) This radiograph of the cervical spine (lateral view) shows evidence of fusion of the apophyseal (facet) joint between C2 and C3 and early signs of enthesitis of the anterior corners of the vertebral bodies, with squaring of anterior corners at the C7/T1 level. (D) This radiograph of the pelvis and thoracolumbar spine (anteroposterior view) shows advanced bilateral sacroiliitis and syndesmophytes in the thoracolumbar spinal junction and an incomplete syndesmophyte arising from the upper left vertebral corner in the lower lumbar spine in a patient with ankylosing spondylitis. (E) This radiograph of the cervical spine (lateral view) shows evidence of prominent anterior complete syndesmophyte between C2 and C3 and fusion of the apophyseal (facet) joints at the same level. (F) This lateral radiographic view of the lumbar spine shows a thick "nonmarginal" syndesmophyte (arising not from the angular margin but from the adjacent anterior surface of the lumbar vertebral body). Such nonmarginal syndesmophytes, often asymmetrical, are seen more often in patients with spondylitis in association with psoriatic or reactive arthritis than in primary ankylosing spondylitis. Reprinted with permission from Elsevier from Khan MA. Ankylosing spondylitis: Clinical features. In Hochberg M, Silman A, Smolen J, Weinblatt M, Weisman M (eds). *Rheumatology* (3rd Ed.). London: Mosby: A Division of Harcourt Health Sciences Ltd.; 2003:1161–1181.

Socioeconomic burden of AS

Ankylosing spondylitis is not an uncommon disease, and it affects men two to three times more commonly than women.[10] Slowly, over many years, the disease results in gradual progressive limitation of spinal mobility and limited chest expansion. It can reduce quality of life and cause severe functional impairment that can result in diminished productivity, work disability, early retirement, and even decreased survival, mostly due to cardiac and pulmonary causes and complications from spinal fracture or surgery.[2,11,12] Patients are less likely to get married, more likely to be divorced, and more than twice as likely to be work-disabled than members of the general population. Women with AS are also less likely to have children than women in the general population.[11]

The burden of this illness has a tremendous impact on the individual patient and society at large, but this burden is largely underestimated. There is a high cost to society resulting from AS due to progressive functional impairment over time. Studies have indicated that indirect costs (those associated with loss of work, etc.) account for nearly 75% of the total costs associated with AS. Since functional disability is the most important predictor of high total costs (both direct medical expenses and indirect costs due to lost wages, reduced productivity, and social function), therapeutic interventions that improve a patient's functional ability will appreciably reduce the overall socioeconomic burden of the disease.[2]

Delay in diagnosis

The clinical presentations of AS can be very heterogeneous, so patients may seek help from various health-care professionals, ranging from their primary care physicians to various medical and surgical specialists, chiropractors, and back pain clinics. Even multiple referrals of such patients to various specialists for their various complaints often do not result in a correct diagnosis. Therefore, unfortunately, many of these patients either are never diagnosed or are inadequately treated, and they experience progressive functional impairment over time.

The diagnosis is often delayed by 5 to 10 years, and during this period many patients undergo unnecessary or even invasive investigations and receive inappropriate treatment.[2,3,13,14] Age at disease onset and at first diagnosis of AS was evaluated by the German AS Society in a survey of 3000 AS patients; the average age of the 1614 respondents (1070 of them men) was 48.8 years (range 20 to 85 years).[13] The distribution curves of age at disease onset (occurrence of initial symptoms) and diagnosis in men and women with AS are shown in Figure 1.3. The first symptoms occurred before the age of 15 years in 4% of the patients, between the ages of 15 and 40 years in 90% of the patients, and after the age of 40 years in 6% of the patients. The average age at disease onset did not differ significantly between men and women. The average delay between disease onset and diagnosis was 8.9 years. There was a longer delay between disease onset and diagnosis in women compared with men (9.8 vs. 8.4 years; $p < 0.01$). In addition to gender, HLA-B27 status also affected the delay in diagnosis; the average delay of diagnosis was 8.5 years in patients with HLA-B27, compared with 11.4 years in patients who lacked HLA-B27 ($p < 0.01$).[14]

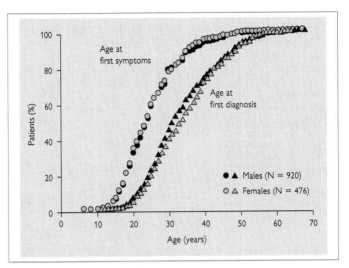

Figure 1.3 Average delay in the diagnosis of ankylosing spondylitis was 8.8 years (8.2 years for males and 9.7 years for females) in this study from Germany. *Source*: Feldtkeller E. Age at disease onset and delayed diagnosis of spondyloarthropathies [German]. *Z Rheumatol*. 1999;58(1):21–30.

   Diagnosing AS at an early stage is not a simple task; one of the difficulties is the nonspecific nature of the disease symptoms in early stages.[9,15] Patients with AS (especially early AS) present most commonly with chronic back pain and stiffness; however, they may underrate these symptoms and may simply adjust to living with them instead of seeking treatment. Also, there are no established criteria for early diagnosis, and many patients have atypical presentations.

Spondyloarthropathies

When AS occurs alone without any associated disease, as is usually the case, it is called primary, uncomplicated, or pure AS; in contrast, secondary AS is accompanied by inflammatory bowel disease (IBD), psoriasis, or reactive arthritis[4,5] (Fig. 1.4). The arthritis observed in AS and in these related diseases is frequently referred to collectively as spondyloarthritis or spondyloarthropathy (SpA) because sacroiliitis, spondylitis, and inflammatory peripheral arthritis are their frequent manifestations.[5] Sometimes the word "seronegative" is added to SpA to denote the lack of association with rheumatoid factor, but this is unnecessary because there is no seropositive form of SpA. Definite classification of the various forms of SpA is not always possible in the early stages of the disease because of their overlapping clinical features, and many patients may be classified as

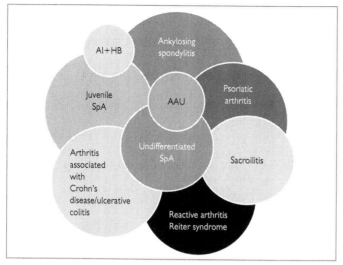

Figure 1.4 This Venn diagram shows the relationships between the spondyloarthropathies. AAU, acute anterior uveitis; AI, aortic incompetence; HB, heart block; SpA, spondyloarthropathies. *Source*: Elyan M, Khan MA. Diagnosing ankylosing spondylitis. *J Rheumatol.* 2006;33(Suppl 78):12–23 (adapted with permission).

having undifferentiated SpA; however, this usually does not affect treatment decisions.

Pharmaceutical interventions in the management of AS

The management of AS challenges and frustrates patients and their families as well as health-care providers. Long-term regular use of nonsteroidal anti-inflammatory drugs (NSAIDs), with a lifelong program of appropriate and regular exercise, has been the first-line treatment and mainstay of symptom control for six decades.[16–18] For patients refractory or intolerant to NSAIDs, various disease-modifying antirheumatic drugs (DMARDs) used for the management of rheumatoid arthritis (RA) are not helpful for treating axial disease; this results in functional impairment and forces many patients to abandon their medical care.

TNF-α antagonists

It is rare that a truly novel and revolutionary therapy becomes available for diseases for which few treatments are effective. This unique phenomenon has finally become a reality for patients with AS with the advent of therapy with tumor necrosis factor-alpha (TNF-α) antagonists, also called biologic response modifiers ("biologicals" for short).[2] TNF-α has been identified as an important mediator of chronic immunoinflammatory disease states, such as RA, AS, psoriasis, ulcerative colitis (UC), and Crohn's disease (CD). The inhibition of TNF-α through a biologically engineered receptor fusion protein (etanercept [Enbrel]) or monoclonal antibodies (infliximab [Remicade], adalimumab [Humira], golimumab) has been shown to markedly decrease inflammatory activity. These TNF-α antagonists are remarkably and equally effective in treating musculoskeletal features of AS, more so than in RA, and do not require any concomitant therapy with conventional DMARDs.[2,19,20]

The monoclonal antibodies (infliximab, adalimumab, and golimumab) and the receptor fusion protein (etanercept) are equally effective in articular manifestation but differ in their efficacy in treating some of the extra-articular manifestations or associated diseases. For example, unlike monoclonal antibodies, etanercept is ineffective in treating UC or CD. In April 2008, certolizumab pegol [Cimzia], a polyethylene glycolated (pegylated) humanized Fab' fragment that binds TNF-α, was approved by the U.S. FDA for the treatment of adult patients with moderate to severe Crohn's disease.

To maintain maximal functional ability, AS patients need to be diagnosed earlier and educated about their disease and about the availability of the new treatment options.[21] Moreover, a lifelong program of appropriate and regular exercise should remain a mainstay of AS treatment, complementing medical therapy.

Historical aspects of AS

AS has affected humans since antiquity; one of the sufferers was the famous Egyptian pharaoh Ramses II. The first skeletal drawing and pathological description of AS was published in 1693 by Bernard Connor (Fig. 1.5). He described an ankylosed skeleton consisting of fused pelvis, spine, and ribs that was unearthed by French farmers in a cemetery. He wrote that the bones were "so straightly and intimately joined, their ligaments perfectly bony, and their articulations so effaced, that they really made but one uniform continuous bone."

The first clinical descriptions of the disease were reported in the mid- to late nineteenth century in a series of publications by Vladimir von Bechterew, Adolf Strümpell, and Pierre Marie. Valentini published the earliest radiographic examination of a patient with AS in 1899, and in 1934 Krebs described the characteristic obliteration of the sacroiliac joints.

The disease has been known by many different names, including spondylitis ankylosans, spondylarthritis ankylopoietica, morbus Bechterew (Bechterew's disease), morbus Strümpell-Marie-Bechterew, and Marie-Strümpell disease. In the past 40 years the term "ankylosing spondylitis" has almost universally been used, but during the first half of the twentieth century the disease was also called rheumatoid spondylitis in some countries, particularly in the United States, because of the erroneous belief that it was just a variant of RA. In 1963 the American Rheumatism Association (the precursor of the American College of Rheumatology) officially adopted

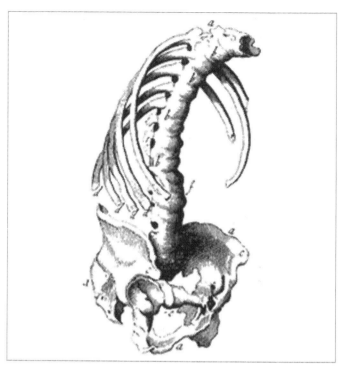

Figure 1.5 This 1695 illustration by Bernard Conner was the first representation of a skeleton of a patient with ankylosing spondylitis. Reprinted with permission from Khan MA. *Ankylosing Spondylitis: The Facts*. Oxford: Oxford University Press; 2002.

the term "ankylosing spondylitis." The concept of SpA was proposed by Moll and Wright in the early 1970s, just before and independent of the discovery in 1973 of the remarkable association of HLA-B27 with this group of diseases.[4,8,22,23]

References

1. Braun J, Sieper J. Ankylosing spondylitis. *Lancet*. 2007;369(9570):1379–1390.

2. Khan MA. Ankylosing spondylitis: burden of illness, diagnosis, and effective treatment. *J Rheumatol Suppl*. 2006;78:1–33.

3. Khan MA. Ankylosing spondylitis: clinical features. In Hochberg M, Silman A, Smolen J, Weinblatt M, Weisman M, eds. *Rheumatology*, 3rd ed. London: Mosby: A Division of Harcourt Health Sciences Ltd.; 2003:1161–1181.

4. Moll JM, Haslock I, Macrae IF, Wright V. Associations between ankylosing spondylitis, psoriatic arthritis, Reiter's disease, the intestinal arthropathies, and Behcet's syndrome. *Medicine (Balt)*. 1974;53(5):343–364.

5. Khan MA. Spondyloarthropathies. In Hunder G, ed. *Atlas of Rheumatology*, 4th ed. Philadelphia: Current Medicine; 2005:151–180.

6. Wellcome Trust Case Control Consortium. Association scan of 14,500 nonsynonymous SNPs in four diseases identifies autoimmunity variants. *Nat Genet.* 2007;39(11):1329–1337.

7. Rahman P. Genetics of ankylosing spondylitis: an update. *Curr Rheumatol Rep.* 2007;9(5):383–389.

8. Khan MA. HLA-B27 and its pathogenic role. *J Clin Rheumatol.* 2008;14(1):50–52.

9. Rudwaleit M, Khan MA, Sieper J. The challenge of diagnosis and classification in early ankylosing spondylitis: do we need new criteria? *Arthritis Rheum.* 2005;52:1000–1008.

10. Akkoc N, Khan MA. Epidemiology of ankylosing spondylitis and related spondyloarthropathies. In Weisman MH, Reveille JD, van der Heijde D, eds. *Ankylosing Spondylitis and the Spondyloarthropathies: A Companion to Rheumatology.* London: Mosby-Elsevier; 2006:117–131.

11. Ward MM, Reveille JD, Learch TJ, Davis JC Jr, Weisman MH. Impact of ankylosing spondylitis on work and family life: comparisons with the US population. *Arthritis Rheum.* 2008;59(4):497–503.

12. Khan MA, Khan MK, Kushner I. Survival among patients with ankylosing spondylitis: a life-table analysis. *J Rheumatol.* 1981;8:86–90.

13. Feldtkeller E. Age at disease onset and delayed diagnosis of spondyloarthropathies [German]. *Z Rheumatol.* 1999;58(1):21–30.

14. Feldtkeller E, Khan MA, van der Linden S, van der Heijde D, Braun J. Age at disease onset and diagnosis delay in HLA-B27 negative vs. positive patients with ankylosing spondylitis. *Rheumatol Int.* 2003;23:61–66.

15. Song JH, Sieper J, Rudwaleit M. Diagnosing early ankylosing spondylitis. *Curr Rheumatol Rep.* 2007;9(5):367–374.

16. Akkoc N, van der Linden S, Khan MA. Ankylosing spondylitis and symptom-modifying vs. disease-modifying therapy. *Best Pract Res Clin Rheumatol.* 2006;20(3):539–557.

17. Elyan M, Khan MA. Does physical therapy have a place in the treatment of ankylosing spondylitis? *Curr Opin Rheumatol.* 2008;20(3):282–286.

18. Sidiropoulos PI, Hatemi G, Song IH, et al. Evidence-based recommendations for the management of ankylosing spondylitis: systematic literature search of the 3E Initiative in Rheumatology involving a broad panel of experts and practising rheumatologists. *Rheumatology (Oxford).* 2008;47(3):355–361.

19. Braun J, Davis J, Dougados M, Sieper J, S vaan der Linden, van der Heijde D, ASAS Working Group. First update of the international ASAS consensus statement for the use of anti-TNF agents in patients with ankylosing spondylitis. *Ann Rheum Dis.* 2006;65(3):316–320.

20. Coates LC, Cawkwell LS, Ng NW, et al. Real life experience confirms sustained response to long-term biologics and switching in ankylosing spondylitis. *Rheumatology (Oxford).* 2008;47(6):897–900.

21. Khan MA. *Ankylosing Spondylitis: The Facts.* Oxford: Oxford University Press; 2002:1–193.

22. Brewerton DA. Discovery: HLA and disease. *Curr Opin Rheumatol.* 2003;15(4):369–373.

23. Khan MA. Five classical clinical papers on ankylosing spondylitis. In Dieppe P, Wollheim FA, Schumacher HR, eds. *Classical Papers in Rheumatology.* London: Martin Dunitz Ltd.; 2002:118–133.

Chapter 2

Epidemiology of ankylosing spondylitis and related spondyloarthropathies

Physicians' perceptions regarding the epidemiology of AS are slowly changing, but numerous misconceptions about AS remain that may contribute to the delay in its diagnosis and effective treatment, including the misperceptions that it is a rare disease and that it is a mild disease that is easy to diagnose.[1-5] According to one study, approximately 5% of chronic back pain sufferers being seen at general practice/primary care practice offices in England "may have a mild form of AS that may never progress to definite ankylosis, but for whom treatment as if they had AS may be of benefit."[6] Early diagnosis of AS is crucial now that more effective therapies are available to suppress disease activity and improve functional ability.[7-9]

For more details on the concepts and epidemiology of AS and related SpA, as well as for the detailed references for the text and the tables in this chapter, the reader is referred to some of the author's publications on the subject.[3,9-12]

Classification criteria

The Rome criteria (1961) were the first set of criteria developed for the classification of AS (Table 2.1). On later evaluation, thoracic pain and uveitis were removed owing to either low specificity or sensitivity, resulting in the New York Classification Criteria (Table 2.2) in 1966. Criteria for chronic inflammatory back pain were proposed in 1977 to help differentiate it from other causes of chronic back pain[13] (Table 2.3).

Modification of the New York criteria was first proposed in 1983,[14,15] incorporating the inflammatory back pain concept,[13] and published a year later.[16] They are now the most widely used criteria to classify AS and are currently (and inappropriately) also being used in clinical practice to establish the diagnosis of AS. According to these criteria, a patient can be classified as having definite AS if at least one clinical criterion (inflammatory back pain, limitation of mobility of the lumbar spine, or limitation of chest expansion) and the radiologic criterion are met (Table 2.4).

Diagnostic criteria for AS have been proposed but have not been properly validated.[7–9,17,18]

Classification criteria for spondyloarthropathies

There are two validated sets of criteria to classify SpA: the European Spondyloarthropathy Study Group (ESSG) criteria (Table 2.5)[19] and the Amor Criteria (Table 2.6).[20] The ESSG criteria are more widely used.

Table 2.1 Rome classification criteria for ankylosing spondylitis

A. Clinical criteria

1. Low back pain and stiffness for >3 months, not relieved by rest
2. Pain and stiffness in the thoracic region
3. Limited motion in the lumbar region
4. Limited chest expansion
5. History of evidence of iritis or its sequelae

B. Radiologic criteria

1. Bilateral sacroiliitis

Definite ankylosing spondylitis is diagnosed if four out of the five clinical criteria are present or bilateral sacroiliitis is associated with any single clinical criterion.

Table 2.2 New York classification criteria for ankylosing spondylitis

A. Clinical criteria

1. Limitation of motion of the lumbar spine in all three planes (anterior flexion, lateral flexion, and extension)
2. A history of pain or the presence of pain at the dorsolumbar junction or in the lumbar spine
3. Limitation of chest expansion to 1 inch (2.5 cm) or less, measured at the level of the fourth intercostal space

B. Radiologic criterion: Sacroiliitis (grading on a 0-to-4 scale)

Normal radiograph of the sacroiliac joints is graded as grade 0

Suspicious changes are grade 1

Minimal abnormality are grade 2

Small areas showing erosion or sclerosis but no alteration in joint width are grade 3

Unequivocal abnormality, moderate or advanced sacroiliitis with erosion(s), sclerosis, widening, narrowing, or partial or complete ankylosis are grade 4

Definite ankylosing spondylitis if:

- Bilateral grade 3 or 4 sacroiliitis in the presence of at least one clinical criterion; or Unilateral grade 3 or 4 or bilateral grade 2 sacroiliitis with clinical criterion 1 or with both clinical criteria 2 and 3

Probable ankylosing spondylitis if:

Bilateral grade 3 or 4 sacroiliitis is present without any clinical criterion.

Table 2.3 Inflammatory-type back pain criteria (Calin)

Inflammatory-type back pain (of AS) is present if there is a clinical history of or current symptoms of spinal pain (in low, middle, and/or upper back, and/or neck region) with at least four of the following five components:

1. At least 3 months duration
2. Onset before age 45
3. Insidious (gradual) onset
4. Improved by exercise
5. Associated with morning spinal stiffness

Table 2.4 Modified New York classification criteria for ankylosing spondylitis

Clinical components

1. Low back pain and stiffness for ≥3 months that improves with exercise but not with rest
2. Limitation of lumbar spine mobility in both the sagittal (sideways) and frontal (forward and backward) planes
3. Limitation in chest expansion as compared with normal range for age and gender

Radiologic component

Unilateral sacroiliitis of grade 3 or 4 or bilateral sacroiliitis of grade ≥2

Diagnosis

1. Definite AS if the radiological criterion is associated with at least one clinical component
2. Probable AS if:
   a. Only the three clinical components are present
      or
   b. Only the radiologic component is present

Table 2.5 European Spondyloarthropathy Study Group criteria

Components	Definition
Inflammatory spinal pain	History of or current symptoms of spinal pain (low, middle, and upper back, or neck region) with at least four of the following five components: 1. At least 3 months in duration 2. Onset before 45 years of age 3. Insidious (gradual) onset 4. Improved by exercise 5. Associated with morning spinal stiffness
Synovitis	Past or present asymmetric arthritis, or arthritis predominately in the lower limbs
Spondyloarthropathy	Presence of inflammatory spinal pain or

Table 2.5 *continued*

Components	Definition
	Synovitis *and* One or more of the following conditions: • Family history: first- or second-degree relatives with ankylosing spondylitis, psoriasis, acute iritis, reactive arthritis, or inflammatory bowel disease • Past or present psoriasis, diagnosed by a physician • Past or present ulcerative colitis or Crohn's disease, diagnosed by a physician and confirmed by radiography or endoscopy • Past or present alternating buttocks pain • Past or present spontaneous pain or tenderness on examination of the site of the insertion of the Achilles tendon or plantar fascia (enthesitis) • Episode of diarrhea occurring within 1 month before onset of arthritis • Nongonococcal urethritis or cervicitis occurring within 1 month before onset of arthritis • Bilateral grade 2 to 4 sacroiliitis or unilateral grade 3 or 4 sacroiliitis according to the following grading system: 0 = normal, 1 = possible, 2 = minimal, 3 = moderate, 4 = completely fused (ankylosed)

Table 2.6 Amor criteria for spondyloarthropathy

Parameters	Scoring
A. Clinical symptoms or past history of:	
1. Lumbar or dorsal pain at night or morning stiffness of lumbar or dorsal region	1
2. Asymmetric oligoarthritis	2
3. Buttock pain	1
	or
Alternating buttock pain	2
4. Sausage-like toe or digit	2
5. Heel pain or other well-defined enthesitis	2
6. Iritis	2
7. Nongonococcal urethritis or cervicitis within 1 month before the onset of arthritis	1
8. Acute diarrhea within 1 month before the onset of arthritis	1
9. Psoriasis, balanitis, or inflammatory bowel disease (ulcerative colitis or Crohn's disease)	2
B. Radiologic findings	
10. Sacroiliitis (bilateral grade 2 or unilateral grade 3)	2
C. Genetic background	
11. Presence of HLA-B27 or family history of AS, reactive arthritis, uveitis, psoriasis, or inflammatory bowel disease	2

Table 2.6 *continued*	
Parameters	Scoring
D. Response to treatment	
12. Clear-cut improvement within 48 hours after NSAID intake or rapid relapse of pain after their discontinuation	2
A patient is considered to be suffering from a spondyloarthropathy if the sum is at least 6.	

Prevalence of AS and related SpA

The prevalence of AS and related SpA has been estimated in several populations using different study designs, such as by screening individuals possessing HLA-B27, most often blood donors or the patients' relatives, by using hospital-based medical records, or by performing population-based surveys in a defined region.[3,12,13] This heterogeneity makes it difficult to compare the prevalence rates obtained in the various studies, and the methodologies used must be carefully evaluated. One may argue that blood donors are unlikely to be representative of the general population. Several hospital-based studies of populations of European extraction have provided prevalence rates that range from 0.1% to 0.8%. However, hospital-based studies may underestimate the true prevalence of AS because they usually reveal only the more severe and typical cases and may not include some patients with mild disease.

Results of population surveys in Europe are shown in Table 2.7. The prevalence rate was found to be high among the population of northern Norway, which has a 16% prevalence of HLA-B27 in the general population. In a very nice epidemiologic study in Tromsø, northern Norway, 14,539 individuals (men age 20 to 54 years and women age 20 to 49) among its 21,329 inhabitants were surveyed for definite AS; the prevalence of AS was 1.1% to 1.4% (1.9% to 2.2% for males and 0.3% to 0.6% for females).[21] It was calculated that 6.7% of the B27-positive individuals and 0.2% of B27-negative individuals had AS, and that 22.5% of the B27-positive subjects with chronic back pain or stiffness had AS.[21]

Few epidemiologic studies have assessed the prevalence of SpA in European populations; the results of those studies are summarized in Table 2.8.

Prevalence studies in the United States

A population-based study from Rochester, Minnesota, covering the years 1935 through 1973 estimated that the point prevalence of AS based on surviving cases was 0.4% in subjects age 45 to 64 years.[22] This figure is clinically more relevant (because it is uncommon for AS to begin after age 45) than the prevalence rate of 0.129% for the general population (1.29 cases per 1000 based on the fact that there were 68 surviving cases of AS among the 52,000 total population of Rochester in 1973).

Table 2.7 Population-based surveys of the prevalence of AS in some European populations, using New York or modified New York criteria

Population	Age	Number studied	Criteria	Prevalence (%)			HLA-B27
				AS			
				Males	Females	Total	
Norway Samis	20 to 62	836	New York	2.7	1	1.8	24
Norway	20 to 49 F 20 to 54 M	14,539	New York	1.9 to 2.2	0.3 to 0.6	1.1 to 1.4	16
Hungary	≥15	6469	New York	0.4	0.08	0.23	13
Greece	≥19	8740	Modified New York	0.4	0.04	0.24	5.4
Turkey	≥20	2835	Modified New York	0.54	0.44	0.49	6.8 to 8.0

Table 2.8 Prevalence of spondyloarthropathies and HLA-B27 in some European populations

Population	Age	Number studied	Diagnosis	Prevalence (%)			HLA-B27
				SpA			
				Males	Females	Total	
France	≥18	2340	Interview/ physical exam	0.41	0.53	0.47	7.5 to 12
Azores	≥50	936	ESSG	2.7	0.4	1.6	
Greece	≥19	8740	ESSG	0.83	0.15	0.49	5.4
Urban/ suburban	≥19	2712/2972	ESSG	1.01/0.91	0.32/0.14	0.65 0.52	
Rural	≥19	3056	ESSG	0.58	0.05	0.32	
Turkey (urban)	≥20	2835	ESSG	0.88	1.22	1.05	6.8

The U.S. National Center for Health Statistics survey report published in 1998 was incomplete and not very robust.[23] In the most recent report published in January 2008, it is estimated that prevalence of AS and related SpA varies from as low as 0.35% (not including undifferentiated SpA) to a highest estimate of 1.3%.[24] This indicates that AS and related SpA affect anywhere between 0.6 million and 2.4 million adults in the United States.[24]

In contrast, rheumatoid arthritis affects only 1.3 million adults, down from the previous estimate of 2.1 million.

Prevalence studies in circumpolar populations

The prevalences of HLA-B27 and AS are high not only among the Samis (Lapps) population of North Norway, as noted above (see Table 2.7), but also among the other native populations of circumpolar Arctic and sub-Arctic regions of Eurasia and North America. Inupiat (Inupiaq) and Yupik Eskimos show a 25% and 40% prevalence of HLA-B27, respectively, and they have a 0.4% prevalence of AS and 2.5% for any form of SpA among adults age 20 and over. Both undifferentiated SpA and reactive arthritis are more common than AS, and HLA-B27 shows a closer association with AS than other spondyloarthropathies.[3,25]

Siberian Chukchis show a 19% to 34% prevalence of HLA-B27, while the Siberian Eskimos, like their North American counterparts, show a 40% prevalence. They have a 0.4% prevalence of AS and 1.5% for any form of SpA.[3,12,13] There is no difference in disease frequency between men and women, but disease appears to be milder in women. HLA-B27 is present in 50% of the general population of Haida Indians living on the Queen Charlotte Islands of British Columbia, Canada, and approximately 10% of adult males in this population have definite AS. Pima Indians, who have an 18% frequency of HLA-B27, have a 2% prevalence of AS among males.[3] Psoriasis and psoriatic arthritis are rare in all of these genetically pure native populations.

Prevalence studies in other populations

Recent population-based epidemiologic studies from Turkey and China have reported a higher prevalence of AS and related SpA than rheumatic arthritis; the prevalence data from Turkey[3,26] are included in Tables 2.7 and 2.8. A recent pooled analysis of 38 epidemiologic studies from China and Taiwan that included 241,169 Han ethnic Chinese adults from 25 provinces or cities found a prevalence range of 0.2% to 0.54% for AS.[27] The prevalence of undifferentiated SpA ranged from 0.64% to 1.2%, and it was 0.01% to 0.1% for psoriatic arthritis and 0.02% for reactive arthritis. Therefore, the overall prevalence of AS and related SpA among the Chinese ranged from 0.87% to 1.84%. In contrast, the prevalence of rheumatoid arthritis ranged from 0.2% to 0.93%, the highest rate being reported from a Taiwan urban area.[27,28]

Conclusion

It has recently been estimated that 0.6 million to 2.4 million adults in the United States have AS and related SpA.[24] In contrast, rheumatoid arthritis affects only 1.3 million adults in the United States, down from the previous estimate of 2.1 million.[24] Recent population-based epidemiologic studies from overseas, primarily from Europe (including Turkey) and China, also indicate a high prevalence of AS and related SpA, much more than previously realized.[3,26–28] All these reports indicate that AS and related diseases as a group are at least as common, if not more common, than rheumatoid arthritis.[3,26–28]

References

1. Rudwaleit M, Khan MA, Sieper J. The challenge of diagnosis and classification in early ankylosing spondylitis: do we need new criteria? *Arthritis Rheum.* 2005;52:1000–1008.

2. Khan MA. Update on spondyloarthropathies. *Ann Intern Med.* 2002; 136:896–907.

3. Akkoc N, Khan MA. Epidemiology of ankylosing spondylitis and related spondyloarthropathies. In Weisman MH, Reveille JD, van der Heijde D, eds. *Ankylosing Spondylitis and the Spondyloarthropathies: A Companion to Rheumatology.* London: Mosby-Elsevier; 2006:117–131.

4. Khan MA. Ankylosing spondylitis: burden of illness, diagnosis, and effective treatment. *J Rheumatol Suppl.* 2006;78:1–33.

5. Khan MA, van der Linden SM, Kushner L, Valkenberg HA, Cats A. Spondylitic disease without radiologic evidence of sacroiliitis in relatives of HLA-B27(+) patients. *Arthritis Rheum.* 1985;28:40–43.

6. Underwood MR, Dawes P. Inflammatory back pain in primary care. *Br J Rheumatol.* 1995;34(11):1074–1077.

7. Khan MA. Thoughts concerning the early diagnosis of ankylosing spondylitis and related diseases. *Clin Exp Rheumatol.* 2002;20(Suppl 28):S6–S10.

8. Rudwaleit M, van der Heijde D, Khan MA, Braun J, Sieper J. How to diagnose axial spondyloarthropathy early. *Ann Rheum Dis.* 2004;63:535–543.

9. Song JH, Sieper J, Rudwaleit M. Diagnosing early ankylosing spondylitis. *Curr Rheumatol Rep.* 2007;9(5):367–374.

10. Sieper J, Rudwaleit M, Khan MA, Braun J. Concepts and epidemiology of spondyloarthritis. *Best Pract Res Clin Rheumatol.* 2006;20(3):401–417.

11. Khan MA. A worldwide overview—the epidemiology of HLA-B27 and associated spondyloarthritides. In Calin A, Taurog J, eds. *The Spondyloarthritides.* Oxford: Oxford University Press; 1998:17–26.

12. Khan MA. Prevalence of HLA-B27 in world populations. In Lopez-Larrea C, ed. *HLA-B27 in the Development of Spondyloarthropathies.* Austin, TX: R.G. Landes Company; 1997:95–112.

13. Calin A, Porta J, Fries JF, Schurman DJ. Clinical history as a screening test for ankylosing spondylitis. *JAMA.* 1977;237(24):2613–2614.

14. van der Linden S, Cats A, Valkenburg HA, Khan MA. Evaluation of the diagnostic criteria for ankylosing spondylitis: a proposal for modification of the New York criteria. *Clin Res.* 1983;31:734A.

15. van der Linden SJ, Cats A, Valkenburg HA, Khan MA. Evaluation of the diagnostic criteria for ankylosing spondylitis: a proposal for modification of the New York criteria. *Br J Rheumatol.* 1984;23:148.

16. van der Linden S, Cats A, Valkenburg HA. Evaluation of diagnostic criteria for ankylosing spondylitis. A proposal for modification of the New York criteria. *Arthritis Rheum.* 1984;27:361–368.

17. Ziedler H, Mau R, Mau W, Freyschmidt J, Majewski A, Deicher H. Evaluation of early diagnostic criteria including HLA-B27 for ankylosing spondylitis in a follow-up study. *Zeitschrift fur Rheumatologie.* 1985;44:249–253.

18. Cats A, van der Linden SM, Goei The HS, Khan MA. Proposals for diagnostic criteria of ankylosing spondylitis and allied disorders. *Clin Exp Rheumatol.* 1987;5:167–171.

19. Dougados M, van der Linden S, Juhlin R, et al. The European Spondylarthropathy Study Group preliminary criteria for the classification of spondylarthropathy. *Arthritis Rheum.* 1991;34(10):1218–1227.

20. Amor B, Dougados M, Mijiyawa M. Criteria of the classification of spondylarthropathies [in French]. *Rev Rhum Mal Osteoartic.* 1990;57(2):85–89.

21. Gran JT, Husby G, Hordvik M. Prevalence of ankylosing spondylitis in males and females in a young middle-aged population of Tromsø, northern Norway. *Ann Rheum Dis.* 1985;44(6):359–367.

22. Carter ET, McKenna CH, Brian DD, Kurland LT. Epidemiology of ankylosing spondylitis in Rochester, Minnesota, 1935–1973. *Arthritis Rheum.* 1979;22(4):365–370.

23. Lawrence RC, Helmick CG, Arnett FC, et al. Estimates of the prevalence of arthritis and selected musculoskeletal disorders in the United States. *Arthritis Rheum.* 1998;41(5):778–799.

24. Helmick CG, Felson DT, Lawrence RC, et al. Estimates of the prevalence of arthritis and other rheumatic conditions in the United States. Part I. *Arthritis Rheum.* 2008;58(1):15–25.

25. Boyer GS, Templin DW, Cornoni-Huntley JC, et al. Prevalence of spondyloarthropathies in Alaskan Eskimos. *J Rheumatol.* 1994;21(12):2292–2297.

26. Onen F, Akar S, Birlik M, et al. Prevalence of ankylosing spondylitis and related spondyloarthritis in an urban area of Izmir, Turkey. *J Rheumatol.* 2008;35(2):305–309.

27. Ng SC, Liao Z, Yu DT, Chan ES, Zhao L, Gu J. Epidemiology of spondyloarthritis in the People's Republic of China: review of the literature and commentary. *Semin Arthritis Rheum.* 2007;37(1):39–47.

28. Akkoc N. Are spondyloarthropathies as common as rheumatoid arthritis? A review. *Curr Rheumatol Rep.* 2008;10:371–378.

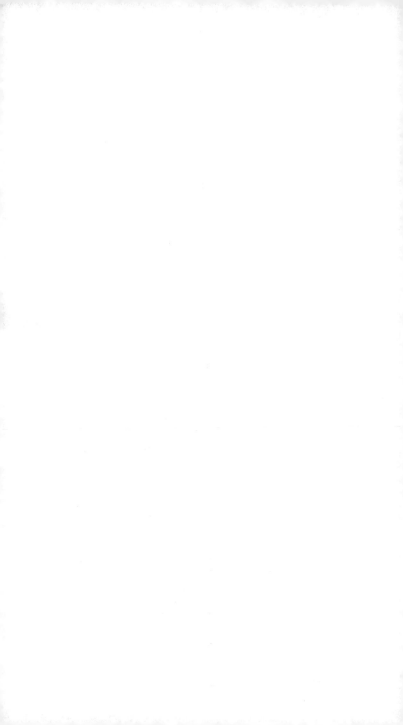

Chapter 3

Causes of ankylosing spondylitis

The precise cause of AS remains unknown, but there is strong evidence that genetic factors play a pivotal role in disease susceptibility, and that they interact with nongenetic (environmental) factors to lead to immune-mediated mechanisms that result in the release of proinflammatory cytokines such as TNF-α.[1–9] More than 90% of the risk of developing AS is determined genetically, indicating the highly heritable nature of this disease.[1–5] There is a strong association with the genetic marker HLA-B27, which lies in the major histocompatibility complex (MHC) region on the short arm of chromosome 6 (6p21 region). However, HLA-B27 is not a prerequisite for AS, as the disease also affects individuals who do not possess HLA-B27.

The recent development of the genome-wide association study approach has revolutionized genetic studies of AS by finding some non-MHC disease genes, some of which also confer susceptibility to Crohn's disease and psoriasis, such as the gene for the interleukin-23 receptor (IL-23R).[1–4] It is of interest that IL-23 is selectively overexpressed in subclinical intestinal inflammation sites in patients with AS at levels similar to those seen in patients with Crohn's disease. IL-23R is a key factor in the regulation of a newly defined proinflammatory effector T-cell subset, Th17 cells.

Successful treatment of psoriasis and Crohn's disease has been reported with a human anti-IL-12p40 monoclonal antibody ustekinumab, which blocks both IL-12 and IL-23, as these cytokines share the IL-12p40 chain.[10,11] Sequence variants in the IL-23R gene and its ligand have also been found to play a role in psoriasis. The IL-23R gene has recently been found to contribute roughly 9% of the population-attributable genetic risk for AS in Caucasians.[1–3] Altogether, these recent findings indicate that genes participating in IL-23 signaling may be a common susceptibility factor for AS, Crohn's disease, and psoriasis by playing a prominent role in the pathogenesis of the chronic epithelial inflammation observed in these diseases.

Another gene, ARTS1 (also called ERAAP and ERAP1), which encodes a transmembrane aminopeptidase with diverse immunologic functions and is located on chromosome 5, shows a strong association with AS, contributing roughly 23% of the population-attributable genetic risk for AS among Caucasian populations.[1,2] ARTS1 is involved in trimming peptides to the optimal length in the endoplasmic reticulum for presentation by MHC class I proteins, and that includes HLA-B27. It also cleaves cell surface receptors for the proinflammatory cytokines IL-1 (IL-1R2), IL-6 (IL-6R-α), and TNF (TNFR1), thereby downregulating their signaling. It is possible that genetic variants of ARTS1 could have proinflammatory effects through this mechanism.

Regions on chromosomes 2 (2p15) and 21 (21q22) also harbor susceptibility genes for AS. One of the members of the IL-1 gene cluster, IL1A, contributes roughly 5% of the population-attributable genetic risk for AS among Caucasian populations.[12] Thus, the population-attributable risks for HLA-B27 (40%), ARTS1 (23%), IL23R (9%), and IL1A (5%) add up, and one can conclude that approximately three-fourths of the total genetic risk of developing AS has been uncovered. These findings may lead to better understanding of the pathogenesis of AS and related SpA and may also provide new therapeutic approaches.

Among the possible environmental triggers for AS onset, infections have long been suspected. It has been speculated that AS may be triggered by gut infection with *Klebsiella* bacteria. However, the evidence is circumstantial, based on the observation by some, but not all, investigators of elevated levels of antibodies against *Klebsiella pneumoniae* in the blood of patients with active disease. More convincing proof has been lacking. Thus, the environmental triggers for AS remain unknown, but the close relationships between AS and psoriasis and clinical and asymptomatic forms of Crohn's disease suggest the potential involvement of an immune reaction in the gut or skin that may be influenced by reactions to microbial infections.

Disease heterogeneity

Heterogeneity of AS has been known for more than 30 years and was first exemplified by the difference between HLA-B27-positive and HLA-B27-negative patients.[13,14] Although there are many similarities, HLA-B27-negative AS is later in its onset; significantly less often complicated by acute anterior uveitis and more frequently accompanied by psoriasis, ulcerative colitis, and Crohn's disease; and less often shows familial aggregation.[13,14] In fact, it is unusual to observe families among people of northern European extraction with two or more first-degree relatives affected with HLA-B27-negative AS in the absence of psoriasis, ulcerative colitis, or Crohn's disease in the family. A recent genetic study supports the existence of an HLA-B27-independent common link between gut inflammation and AS.[9]

Individuals who are homozygous for HLA-B27 are more than three times as likely to get the disease as those who are heterozygotes.[15] This has recently been confirmed in a study from Finland.[16] There are many possible explanations for this observation. These include, for example, possible increased cell surface expression of HLA-B27 or potentially increased effect of linked genes that may have influence on disease process occurrence.

Hypotheses to explain the pathogenic role of HLA-B27

The precise explanation for the association of HLA-B27 and AS, one of the strongest between an MHC molecule and a disease, has eluded researchers for more than 35 years. HLA-B27 is the primary disease susceptibility gene for AS, contributing roughly 40% of the population-attributable genetic risk of AS in Caucasians.[1,2]

Several hypotheses have been proposed that are based on the fact that the HLA-B27 molecule, besides having its peptide-presenting specificity, folds slowly, tends to misfold, and can form covalent heavy chain homodimers amenable to recognition by leukocyte receptors that might predispose to disease through immunomodulation of both innate and adaptive responses to arthritogenic pathogens.[5–8] But none of the proposed theories has as yet satisfactorily explained the underlying mechanism and the differential association of HLA-B27 subtypes with AS. There are more than 52 subtypes (alleles) of HLA-B27 based on nucleotide sequence differences, but at the translated protein level the number of subtypes ranges from HLA-B*2701 to HLA-B*2743. The common subtypes B*2702, B*2704, and B*2705 are strongly associated with AS. Among the other subtypes, most of which are relatively uncommon, B*2701, B*2703, B*2707, B*2708, B*2714, B*2715, and B*2719 are known to be disease associated (or, at least, AS patients possessing these subtypes have been observed). B*2706, a subtype occurring in southeast Asia, does not predispose to AS, and this may also be the case with B*2709, a rare subtype primarily observed among Italians living on the island of Sardinia.[5–8,17]

According to the "arthritogenic peptide" hypothesis, there must be one or more arthritogenic peptides for AS, but none has been found. This hypothesis suggests that the ability of HLA-B27 to bind such a peptide or a set of peptides, either microbial or self-derived, results in disease from an HLA-B27-restricted CD8+ cytotoxic T-cell response to such peptides found only in affected sites.[8] Such a peptide could be bound and presented by all disease-associated subtypes of HLA-B27 but not by other HLA class I molecules. It was originally thought that if there is an arthritogenic peptide, the CD8+ T cells would play a role, because MHC restriction dictates that CD8+ T cells conventionally interact with MHC class I molecules, while CD4+ T cells interact with MHC class II molecules. But evidence is mounting that the CD8+ T cells may not be the cells that are involved, at least in the B27 transgenic mouse model for SpA that has been studied.

Patients with AS who possess a disease-associated subtype of HLA-B27 called B*2705 carry precursor T cells specific for a well-defined self peptide (from the vasoactive intestinal peptide receptor 1, pVIPR). In contrast, individuals possessing B*2709, a subtype not associated with AS, lacked such a reactivity. X-ray crystallography has shown that the B*2705 binds the pVIPR peptide in two distinct conformations, whereas the B*2709 molecule presents the same peptide in only one of the two conformations. This suggests that the dual conformation of the peptide in the B*2705 molecules could result in a less efficient negative selection in B*2705-positive individuals.[5–8]

Data from a viral peptide derived from the Epstein-Barr virus suggest that molecular mimicry between a viral-derived and a self-derived peptide could trigger a cross-reactive cytotoxic T-cell response activating the clonotypes that have not been eliminated during ontogenesis in the thymus.

This failure to eliminate the self-peptide-activated T cells during development may contribute to the autoimmune and inflammatory process in later years in AS patients.[5–8]

HLA-B27, like the other MHC class I molecules, is made up of a heavy chain and a light (β-2 microglobin) chain. The two chains can dissociate, allowing the heavy chain to covalently attach to another heavy chain to form heavy chain homodimers on the cell surface that are amenable to recognition by leukocyte receptors, leading to pathogenic immune responses. In the past few years the research focus has shifted from the peptide-presenting function of HLA-B27 to include ideas based on aberrant aspects of its immunobiology.[5–8,17] There is a growing interest in the abnormal processing and folding of endogenous proteins playing a role in the pathogenesis in many diseases. An excess of misfolded HLA-B27 proteins in the endoplasmic reticulum may activate an unfolded-protein response that can trigger inflammation. Recently, in a rat model of spondyloarthropathies, an activation of the unfolded-protein response in macrophages has been reported to correlate with the inflammatory disease.[18]

Another hypothesis proposes that HLA-B27 itself becomes autoantigenic due to its sequence homology with certain bacterial proteins.[8] Lastly, it has been proposed that B27 may modify intracellular microbial-handling putative arthritogenic organisms that can result in an aberrant or impaired immune response that leads to AS or related SpA.[8] It is even possible that HLA-B27 may predispose to AS via more than one mechanism, or by different mechanisms in different patients, based on additional genetic and nongenetic factors.

References

1. Brown MA. Breakthroughs in genetic studies of ankylosing spondylitis. *Rheumatology (Oxford)*. 2008;47(2):132–137.

2. Wellcome Trust Case Control Consortium, et al. Association scan of 14,500 nonsynonymous SNPs in four diseases identifies autoimmunity variants. *Nat Genet*. 2007;39(11):1329–1337.

3. Rahman P. Genetics of ankylosing spondylitis: an update. *Curr Rheumatol Rep*. 2007;9(5):383–389.

4. Rahman P, Inman RD, Gladman DD, Reeve JP, Peddle L, Maksymowych WP. Association of interleukin-23 receptor variants with ankylosing spondylitis. *Arthritis Rheum*. 2008;58(4):1020–1025.

5. Khan MA, Mathieu A, Sorrentino R, Akkoc N. The pathogenetic role of HLA-B27 and its subtypes. *Autoimmun Rev*. 2007;6(3):183–189.

6. Khan MA. HLA-B27 and its pathogenic role. *J Clin Rheumatol*. 2008;14(1):50–52.

7. Taurog J. The mystery of HLA-B27: if it isn't one thing, it's another. *Arthritis Rheum*. 2007;56(8):2478–2481.

8. Marcilla M, de Castro JA. Peptides: the cornerstone of HLA-B27 biology and pathogenetic role in spondyloarthritis. *Tissue Antigens*. 2008;71(6):495–506.

9. Thjodleifsson B, Geirsson AJ, Björnsson S, Bjarnason I. A common genetic background for inflammatory bowel disease and ankylosing spondylitis: a genealogic study in Iceland. *Arthritis Rheum*. 2007;56(8):2633–2639.

10. Papp KA, Langley RG, Lebwohl M, et al. Efficacy and safety of ustekinumab, a human interleukin-12/23 monoclonal antibody, in patients with psoriasis: 52-week results from a randomised, double-blind, placebo-controlled trial (PHOENIX 2). *Lancet.* 2008; 371:1675–1684.

11. Fuss IJ, Becker C, Yang Z, et al. Both IL-12p70 and IL-23 are synthesized during active Crohn's disease and are down-regulated by treatment with anti-IL-12 p40 monoclonal antibody. *Inflamm Bowel Dis.* 2006;12(1):9–15.

12. Sims AM, Timms AE, Bruges-Armas J, et al. Prospective meta-analysis of IL-1 gene complex polymorphisms confirms associations with ankylosing spondylitis. *Ann Rheum Dis.* 2008 March 4 [E-pub ahead of print].

13. Khan MA, Kushner I, Braun WE. Comparison of clinical features of HLA-B27 positive and negative patients with ankylosing spondylitis. *Arthritis Rheum.* 1977;20:909–912.

14. Khan MA, Kushner I, Braun WE. Genetic heterogeneity in primary ankylosing spondylitis. *J Rheumatol.* 1980;7:383–386.

15. Khan MA, Kushner I, Braun WE, Zachary AA, Steinberg AG. HLA-B27 homozygosity in ankylosing spondylitis: relationship to risk and severity. *Tissue Antigens.* 1978;11:434–438.

16. Jaakkola E, Herzberg J, Laiho K, et al. Finnish HLA studies confirm the increased risk conferred by HLA-B27 homozygosity in ankylosing spondylitis. *Ann Rheum Dis.* 2006;65(6):775–780.

17. Khan MA. Recent advances in the genetics of ankylosing spondylitis. *Future Rheumatology.* 2008 (in press).

18. Turner MJ, Delay ML, Bai S, Klenk E, Colbert RA. HLA-B27 up-regulation causes accumulation of misfolded heavy chains and correlates with the magnitude of the unfolded protein response in transgenic rats: implications for the pathogenesis of spondylarthritis-like disease. *Arthritis Rheum.* 2007;56(1):215–223.

Chapter 4

Disease process

As stated earlier, enthesitis (painful inflammation of entheses) is an important and characteristic clinicopathologic feature of AS and related SpA, but it is not the sole feature.[1] Synovitis and subchondral bone marrow changes adjacent to the ligamentous insertions are important too, as are cartilage proliferation and endochondral ossification. But entheses may also be affected by metabolic, degenerative, and mechanical factors that can result in noninflammatory pathology, termed *enthesopathy* (Table 4.1).[1–5]

The entheseal insertions are ubiquitous, and therefore a variety of anatomic sites can be symptomatically involved in SpA due to widespread enthesitis (Table 4.2). The pathologic lesion starts with soft tissue inflammation, followed by the underlying bone marrow "edema" (osteitis) with only occasional inflammatory cells. These changes predate the bone cortex erosion and new bone formation. Enthesitis occurs mostly at various well-defined locations; these are predominantly in the axial skeleton (including

Table 4.1 Causes of enthesitis/enthesopathy

Inflammatory causes (enthesitis)

Ankylosing spondylitis

Reactive arthritis/Reiter's syndrome

Psoriatic arthritis

Enteropathic arthritis/inflammatory bowel disease

Juvenile spondyloarthropathy/late-onset pauciarticular juvenile arthritis

Undifferentiated spondyloarthropathy

Noninflammatory causes (enthesopathy)

Mechanical/degenerative

Trauma

Osteoarthritis

Metabolic/endocrine/idiopathic enthesopathy

Diffuse idiopathic skeletal hyperostosis (Forestier's disease)

Acromegaly

Fluorosis

Retinoid therapy

Hypoparathyroidism

Hyperparathyroidism

X-linked hypophosphatemia

POEMS syndrome

Miscellaneous

Lyme disease

Leprosy

Table 4.2 Entheseal structures most frequently involved in AS and related SpA

Axial skeleton (including sacroiliac, hip, and shoulder joints)

Pelvic bones: iliac crest, gluteal (ischial) tuberosity, pubic symphysis

Anterior chest wall

Achilles tendon

Plantar fascia

Insertion of supraspinous tendon

Tibial tuberosity

Greater femoral trochanter

several pelvic sites and the chest wall) and the lower extremities. These sites include the trochanteric regions of the femur and the insertions of the Achilles tendon and plantar aponeurosis (into the calcaneum) and the patellar tendon (into the tibial tubercle of the knee).[2–5]

There are two types of entheses: the fibrous type (on membranous bone) and the fibrocartilaginous type (on endochondral bone, such as the insertion of the supraspinatus tendon into the upper surface of the humeral head). The fibrous type of enthesis is characterized by pure dense fibrous connective tissue that attaches the tendon or ligament to the bone, while the fibrocartilaginous type is characterized by a transitional zone of fibrocartilage at the bony interface. Fibrous entheses are typical of the metaphyses and diaphyses of long bones (e.g., insertion of deltoid muscle into the shaft of the humerus), but most entheses are fibrocartilaginous (e.g., the sites of tendon insertions into the epiphyses of long bones). Fibrocartilage is most typical of tendons and ligaments where the angle of attachment changes throughout the range of joint movement (e.g., insertion of the supraspinatus muscle into the top of the humerus).

The fibrocartilaginous enthesis has four components:

1. compact fiber bundles region,
2. a zone of uncalcified (nonmineralized) fibrocartilage where the cell morphology changes to that of chondrocytes,
3. An abrupt transition to calcified (mineralized) fibrocartilage
4. Lamellar bone

The nonmineralized fibrocartilage is structurally, chemically, and biomechanically intermediate between tendon and cartilage. The sites where synovial joint capsules insert into the bone can also be regarded as an enthesis containing fibrocartilage, and I have suggested that we need to broaden the concept of enthesis even further to include the sites of the hyaline and/or fibrocartilage attachments at the ends of the bones.[2] This proposal would imply that the chondral–subchondral junction of bone where cartilage, rather than exclusively ligament/tendon, attaches to the bone should also be regarded as an enthesis. The enthesis as defined by me[2] is the primary site of involvement; this is supported by histopathologic findings and recent MRI studies in which patients with early AS and related SpA often show inflammatory subchondral bone changes (Fig. 4.1).[6–9]

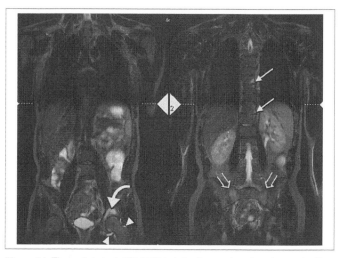

Figure 4.1 These whole-body MRI (STIR technique) coronal sections show enthesitis in the spine, sacroiliac joints, and left hip joint. The curved arrow shows involvement with subchondral bone edema (osteitis), and the arrowheads point to effusion in the left hip joint. The straight arrows point to corner lesions indicating enthesitis in the spine, and the open arrows point to bilateral sacroiliitis. Reprinted, with permission from Remedica Medical Education and Publishing, from Weber U, Pfirrmann CWA, Khan MA. Ankylosing spondylitis: update on imaging and therapy. *Int J Adv Rheumatol.* 2007;5(1):2–7.

Combined MRI and ultrasonographic studies suggest that entheseal soft tissue abnormalities may predate the onset of bone edema. The inflammation may spontaneously resolve and recur, or migrate to other sites of bone-cartilage interface,[9] and the synovium may not be the primary target organ in AS and related SpA. In contrast to rheumatoid arthritis, where structural damage occurs in only two steps (inflammation followed by erosive bone destruction), the histopathologic findings in AS suggest that the structural damage in this disease happens in three steps:[9]

1. Chronic inflammation, the first step, leads to infiltration of subchondral tissues and bone (osteitis) by plasma cells, lymphocytes, mast cells, macrophages, and chondrocytes. Affected sites show irregular erosions of cartilage and adjacent bone. This inflammatory granulation tissue in the spine usually begins at the junction of the annulus fibrosus and the corners of the vertebral body, and can be seen on MRI T2-weighted or STIR images as characteristic shiny corners.
2. This is followed by repair of these lesions by mostly fibrous tissue and fibrocartilage, and remodeling and some reactive bone sclerosis.
3. In the final step of osteoproliferation, the healing tissue gradually becomes ossified, and the affected sites such as the sacroiliac and facet joints gradually become fused. The same process affects the outer layers of the annulus fibrosus in the affected region of the spine, and it is slowly replaced by bony bridging (syndesmophytes).

This osteoproliferation and resultant fusion usually first begin in the mid- and lower thoracic and upper lumbar spine and may extend to involve the whole spine, resulting in "bamboo spine" in severe cases of long-standing disease. This bony fusion is a slowly evolving process that takes place over many months and years. Presence of a syndesmophyte is the best predictor of the subsequent appearance of new syndesmophytes at other sites.

Inflammation and osteoproliferation

There is evidence that TNF-α, a proinflammatory cytokine, plays a pivotal role in the inflammatory cascade of AS, perhaps more so than in rheumatoid arthritis.[9] High amounts of TNF messenger RNA and protein have been detected in the sacroiliac joint tissue of patients with AS. TNF-α levels are higher in the serum of AS patients than in patients with noninflammatory back pain. Significantly higher levels of TNF-α are also found in the affected joints of AS patients.

TNF-α and other cytokines, such as interleukin (IL)-1 and IL-17, are potent inducers of osteoclast formation, either by direct stimulation of these cells or by inducing the expression of RANKL (receptor activator of nuclear factor-kappaB ligand), a critical mediator for bone resorption in arthritis.[10] However, joints have a natural "response to stress" mechanism that can result in new bone formation, such as osteophytes. This reaction is also abundant in AS and related SpA, but it is virtually absent in RA. Recent data indicate that inflammation itself inhibits osteoproliferation via TNF-α and Dickkopf-1 (DKK-1), a regulatory molecule of the Wingless protein (Wnt) pathway.[10–12] DKK-1 inhibits Wnt-mediated proliferation and differentiation of osteoblasts TNF-α causes bone resorption by inducing the expression of DKK-1. Thus, blockade of either TNF-α or DKK-1 in a mouse model of inflammatory arthritis reverses the bone-destructive pattern into a bone-forming pattern.

TNF blockers target sites of active inflammation but do not directly inhibit osteoproliferation, so it is not surprising that, in an animal model of joint ankylosis, etanercept failed to inhibit osteoproliferation.[12,13] There is a need to study a large number of AS patients with early disease and treat them for a longer period of time to establish whether TNF antagonists do or do not inhibit syndesmophyte formation. In the meantime, AS patients taking TNF antagonists should, if possible, not taper off their NSAIDs because there is evidence that the NSAIDs do to some extent inhibit osteoproliferation, possibly by inhibiting prostaglandins (see Chapter 12).

The following recent findings may help in the development of new therapeutic targets in the future:[8–12]

- The Wnt pathway regulates osteoblastic bone formation and remodeling in inflammatory arthritis.
- DKK-1 is a master regulator of joint remodeling; it inhibits Wnt-mediated proliferation and differentiation of osteoblasts. DKK-1 levels are low

in patients with AS (unlike rheumatoid arthritis); this may explain the excessive new bone formation in AS.

- TNF-α induces DKK-1 production by synoviocytes.
- TNF antagonists suppress DKK-1 production.
- This may explain why in AS TNF antagonists have the ability to suppress inflammation but may not prevent radiographic progression; however, long-term studies are needed to confirm or refute this possibility.[9,13,14]

Autoinflammatory syndromes

The term "autoinflammatory syndromes," originally used for clinically defined hereditary periodic fever syndromes, including familial Mediterranean fever and TNF receptor–associated periodic syndrome, has recently been used to describe a distinct group of systemic inflammatory diseases that are apparently not infectious, autoimmune, allergic, or immunodeficient in etiology; are caused by or associated with mutations of genes regulating innate immunity; and have common clinical features accompanied by activation of neutrophils and/or monocytes/macrophages. It is a self-directed inflammation in which local factors at sites predisposed to disease lead to activation of innate immune cells, including macrophages and neutrophils, with resultant target tissue damage.[15,16] Such a dysregulation of innate immune signaling seems to play a role also in diseases such as Crohn's disease, ulcerative colitis, psoriasis and psoriatic arthritis, and possibly other forms of SpA.

References

1. McGonagle D, Khan MA, Marzo-Ortega H, O'Connor P, Gibbon W, Emery P. Enthesitis in spondyloarthropathy. *Curr Opin Rheumatol.* 1999;11:244–250.
2. Khan MA. Enthesitis: a broader definition. *Ann Rheum Dis.* 2000;59:998.
3. François RJ, Braun J, Khan MA. Entheses and enthesitis: a histopathologic review and relevance to spondyloarthritides. *Curr Opin Rheumatol.* 2001;13(4):255–264.
4. Braun J, Khan MA, Sieper J. Entheses and enthesopathy: what is the target of the immune response? *Ann Rheum Dis.* 2000;59:985–994.
5. McGonagle D, Gibbon W, Emery P. Classification of inflammatory arthritis by enthesitis. *Lancet.* 1998;352:1137–1140
6. Olivieri I, Barozzi L, Padula A. Enthesiopathy: clinical manifestations, imaging and treatment. *Baillieres Clin Rheumatol.* 1998;12:665–681.
7. McGonagle D, Gibbon W, O'Connor P, Green M, Pease C, Emery P. Characteristic MRI entheseal changes of knee synovitis in spondyloarthropathy. *Arthritis Rheum.* 1998;41:694–700.
8. Eshed I, Bollow M, McGonagle D, et al. MRI of enthesitis of the appendicular skeleton in spondyloarthritis. *Ann Rheum Dis.* 2007;66:1553–1559.
9. Appel H, Sieper J. Spondyloarthritis at the crossroads of imaging pathology and structural damage in the era of biologics. *Curr Rheumatol Rep.* 2008;10:356–363.
10. Diarra D, Stolina M, Polzer K, et al. Inflammation and destruction of the joints—the Wnt pathway. *Joint Bone Spine.* 2008;75(2):105–107.

11. Diarra D, Stolina M, Polzer K, et al. Dickkopf-1 is a master regulator of joint remodeling. *Nat Med.* 2007; 13(2):156–163.

12. Schett G, Landewé R, van der Heijde D. Tumour necrosis factor blockers and structural remodelling in ankylosing spondylitis: what is reality and what is fiction? *Ann Rheum Dis.* 2007;66:709–711.

13. Sieper J, Appel H, Braun J, Rudwaleit M. Critical appraisal of assessment of structural damage in ankylosing spondylitis: implications for treatment outcomes. *Arthritis Rheum.* 2008;58(3):649–656.

14. Baraliakos X, Listing J, Brandt J, et al. Radiographic progression in patients with ankylosing spondylitis after 4 yrs of treatment with the anti-TNF-alpha antibody infliximab. *Rheumatology (Oxford).* 2007;46(9):1450–1453.

15. McGonagle D, Tan AL, Benjamin M. The biomechanical link between skin and joint disease in psoriasis and psoriatic arthritis: what every dermatologist needs to know. *Ann Rheum Dis.* 2008;67:1–4.

16. McGonagle D, McDermott MF. A proposed classification of the immunological diseases. *PLoS Med.* 2006;3(8):e297.

Chapter 5

Clinical features

The clinical features of AS are very heterogeneous; they can be divided into musculoskeletal and extraskeletal manifestations (Table 5.1). The disease symptoms usually start insidiously when patients are in their late teens or early 20s; males are affected roughly twice as commonly as females. Data from developed countries indicate that the average age of onset is around 24 years; onset before age 10 or after age 45 is rare. Approximately 15% of patients have onset of their disease in childhood (before age 16), but this percentage may be as high as 40% in some developing countries.[1–3]

Chronic low back pain and stiffness

The most common and characteristic initial symptoms are chronic low back pain and stiffness, usually of insidious onset and dull in character. However, many patients complain of pain in the buttock region as their earliest symptom; it may be unilateral or intermittent at first, or may alternate, appearing first in one buttock and then the other, but it generally becomes persistent and bilateral within a few months.[1–10] The pain resulting from sacroiliac joint inflammation is difficult to localize by the patient and is felt deep in the gluteal region. Some patients may note radiation of pain down the upper part of the posterior thigh region, which can be misdiagnosed as lumbago or sciatica, even though the results of the neurologic examination are within normal limits.[1] These symptoms may be accompanied by sacroiliac or spinal tenderness.

Back symptoms tend to worsen after prolonged periods of inactivity ("gel phenomenon") and are therefore worse in the morning. The pain and

Table 5.1 Clinical spectrum of AS	
Musculoskeletal	Axial arthritis (e.g., sacroiliitis and spondylitis)
	Arthritis of girdle joints (hips and shoulders)
	Peripheral arthritis
	Others: enthesitis, osteoporosis, vertebral fractures, spondylodiscitis, pseudarthrosis
Extraskeletal	Acute anterior uveitis
	Cardiovascular involvement
	Pulmonary involvement
	Cauda equina syndrome
	Enteric mucosal lesions
	Miscellaneous, such as amyloidosis

stiffness tend to be eased by moving about (limbering up), with physical activity or exercise, or by a hot shower. Some patients may wake up at night to exercise or move about for a few minutes before returning to bed. The patient often has difficulty getting out of bed because of pain and stiffness and may roll sideways off the bed, trying not to flex or rotate the spine. The back pain and stiffness can be quite severe at this early stage, and the pain tends to be accentuated with coughing, sneezing, or maneuvers that cause a sudden twist of the back.[1]

Because of the high prevalence of back pain in the population at large, it is helpful to elicit from the clinical history certain features that differentiate the noninflammatory causes from the inflammatory back pain of AS and related SpA.[4]

Characteristically, the onset of inflammatory back symptoms is insidious rather than abrupt, and the patient often cannot precisely date the onset of symptoms because they may have been trivial or fleeting aches and pains in the beginning. As the symptoms become chronic (defined as persistence for at least 3 months), the patient notices prominent back pain and stiffness in the morning that usually last for half an hour or more. The symptoms improve with physical activity or exercise but not with rest. They get worse after prolonged rest, such as during the second half of the night and the early morning hours, and may interrupt sleep. Therefore, inadequate sleep and daytime somnolence and fatigue can be major complaints.[1]

Spondylitis starts in its earliest stage (pre-radiographic) with symptoms of inflammatory back pain. To better define the features of inflammatory back pain, Rudwaleit et al.[5] compared the clinical history of 101 patients with AS with that of 112 patients with mechanical (ubiquitous) low back pain. All the patients were less than 50 years of age and had chronic (>3 months) back pain. The researchers came up with the modified criteria for inflammatory back pain: morning stiffness for at least 30 minutes, stiffness improved by exercise but not rest, awakening because of back pain during the second half of the night, and alternating buttock pain (Table 5.2). If the patient has chronic back pain that began before age 50, the presence of any two of these four parameters indicates the presence of inflammatory back pain with a sensitivity of 70.3% and a specificity of 81.2%.[5]

Sometimes pain and stiffness in the midthoracic or the cervical region or chest pain may be the initial symptom, rather than the more typical low backache.[7–9] This may be a relatively more common presentation in

---

Table 5.2 New criteria for inflammatory-type back pain

In a patient with chronic back pain (>3 months) with onset before age 50 years, inflammatory-type back pain (IBP) is present with a sensitivity of 70.3% and a specificity of 81.2% if any two of the following four criteria are fulfilled:

1. Morning stiffness for >30 minutes
2. Improvement in back pain with exercise but not with rest
3. Awakening because of back pain during the second half of the night only
4. Alternating buttock pain

women than in men. Generally the pain and stiffness in the cervical spine evolve after some years but occasionally occur in the early stages of the disease, and some patients may have recurrent severe episodes of stiff neck (torticollis).[1,10]

Other clinical presentations

Occasionally, back pain may be absent or too mild to impel the patient to seek medical care. Some patients may complain only of back stiffness, fleeting muscle aches, or musculotendinous tender spots. These symptoms may become worse on exposure to cold or dampness, and some of these patients may be misdiagnosed with fibromyalgia.[1] Mild constitutional symptoms, such as anorexia, malaise, weight loss, and low-grade fever, may occur in some patients in the early stages of the disease; these are more common among patients with juvenile-onset AS, especially in developing countries.[1] In many patients, daytime fatigue and getting tired easily as well as sleep disturbance are major complaints. Many patients complain of lack of adequate uninterrupted sleep because of back pain and stiffness that is worse at night. In a study of AS patients, too little sleep was reported by approximately 80% of the female and 50% of the male patients, compared to less than 29% and 22%, respectively, in the general population.[11]

Clinical presentations due to enthesitis, peripheral arthritis, or acute anterior uveitis may sometimes antedate or accompany back symptoms. Enthesitis resulting in extraarticular or juxtaarticular bony tenderness can be a major or presenting complaint in some patients, especially among those with juvenile-onset AS. It may appear alone or with arthritis and can cause tenderness of the costosternal junctions, spinous processes, iliac crests, greater femoral trochanters, ischial tuberosities, tibial tubercles, or the sites of attachments of ligaments and tendons to the calcaneus and tarsal bones of the feet. Plantar fasciitis and Achilles tendinitis can result in heel pain and tenderness over the inferior and posterior surfaces of the calcaneus, respectively.[1]

Involvement of the thoracic spine (including the costovertebral and costotransverse joints) and anterior chest wall (costosternal enthesitis and inflammation of the manubriosternal junction (Fig. 5.1) or sternoclavicular joints) may cause chest pain that may be the initial complaint.[1,12] Many patients give a history of having complained to their physicians about chest pain before AS was diagnosed. The chest pain is accentuated on coughing or sneezing and at times may even mimic symptoms of atypical angina or pericarditis. Some patients notice an inability to expand the chest fully on inspiration.

Sometimes the first symptoms may result from involvement of "root" or "girdle" joints (the hips and the shoulders). Hip joint involvement has been correlated with early age at onset of AS and is an indicator for a bad prognosis. Involvement of peripheral joints other than the hips and shoulders is uncommon in primary AS in developed countries, although the sites affected may include the knees, wrists, elbows, and feet. When present,

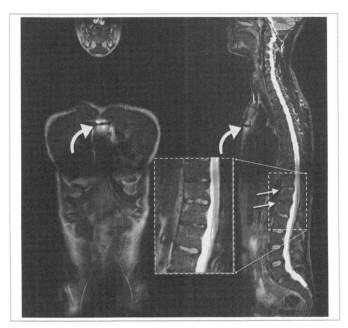

Figure 5.1 These whole-body MRI (STIR technique) coronal and sagittal sections show manubrial involvement in a patient with ankylosing spondylitis. Curved arrows indicate involvement of the manubriosternal joint, and straight arrows point to corner lesions (enthesis) in the spine. Reprinted, with permission from Remedica Medical Education and Publishing, from Weber U, Pfirrmann CWA, Khan MA. Ankylosing spondylitis: update on imaging and therapy. *Int J Adv Rheumatol.* 2007:5(1):2–7.

involvement is usually asymmetric, monoarticular, or oligoarticular; it is normally mild and rarely persistent or erosive and resolves without any residual joint deformity in most patients. Enthesitis of the extremities and peripheral joint involvement are relatively more common in developing countries and also among patients who have associated psoriasis or inflammatory bowel disease, or those with juvenile-onset AS.[13] MRI, especially the new whole body MRI, can be very helpful in making an early diagnosis in such patients.[14,15] Peripheral joint involvement occasionally occurs after the axial disease has become inactive.

References

1. Khan MA. Ankylosing spondylitis: clinical features. In Hochberg M, Silman A, Smolen J, Weinblatt M, Weisman M, eds. *Rheumatology*, 3rd ed. London: Mosby: A Division of Harcourt Health Sciences Ltd.; 2003:1161–1181.

2. Khan MA. Update on spondyloarthropathies. *Ann Intern Med.* 2002;136:896–907.

3. Khan MA. Spondyloarthropathies. In Hunder G, ed. *Atlas of Rheumatology*, 4th ed. Philadelphia: Current Medicine; 2005:151–180.

4. Sieper J, van der Heijde D, Landewé R, et al. Inflammatory back pain criteria according to experts—a real patient exercise by the Assessment in Spondyloarthritis International Society (ASAS). *Ann Rheum Dis* (in press).

5. Rudwaleit M, Metter A, Listing J, Sieper J, Braun J. Inflammatory back pain in ankylosing spondylitis: a reassessment of the clinical history for application as classification and diagnostic criteria. *Arthritis Rheum*. 2006;54(2):569–578.

6. Khan MA. Thoughts concerning the early diagnosis of ankylosing spondylitis and related diseases. *Clin Exp Rheumatol*. 2002;20(Suppl 28):S6–S10.

7. Rudwaleit M, Khan MA, Sieper J. How to diagnose axial SpA early. *Ann Rheum Dis*. 2004;63:535–543.

8. Khan MA, van der Linden SM, Kushner I, Valkenburg HA, Cats A. Spondylitic disease without radiological evidence of sacroiliitis in relatives of HLA-B27(+) patients. *Arthritis Rheum*. 1985;28:40–43.

9. Rudwaleit M, Khan MA, Sieper J. The challenge of diagnosis and classification in early ankylosing spondylitis: do we need new criteria? *Arthritis Rheum*. 2005;52:1000–1008.

10. Weber U, Pfirrmann CWA, Kissling RO, MacKenzie CR, Khan MA. Early spondyloarthritis in HLA-B27 positive monozygotic twin pair: a highly concordant onset, sites of involvement, and disease course. *J Rheumatol*. 2008;35(7):1464–1467.

11. Hultgren S, Broman JE, Gudbjörnsson B, Hetta J, Lindqvist U. Sleep disturbances in outpatients with ankylosing spondylitis: a questionnaire study with gender implications. *Scand J Rheumatol*. 2000;29(6):365–369.

12. van der Linden SM, Khan MA, Rentsch H-U, et al. Chest pain without radiographic sacroiliitis in relatives of patients with ankylosing spondylitis. *J Rheumatol*. 1988;15:836–839.

13. O'Shea FD, Boyle E, Riarh R, Tse SM, Laxer RM, Inman RD. Comparison of clinical and radiographic severity of juvenile-onset versus adult-onset ankylosing spondylitis. *Ann Rheum Dis*. 2008 Sep 9 [Epub ahead of print].

14. Song IH, Sieper J, Rudwaleit M. Diagnosing early ankylosing spondylitis. *Curr Rheumatol Rep*. 2007;9(5):367–374.

15. Weber U, Kissling JO, Hodler J. Advances in musculoskeletal imaging and their clinical utility in the early diagnosis of spondyloarthritis. *Curr Rheumatol Rep*. 2007;9(5):353–360.

Chapter 6

Physical findings

Clinical signs are sometimes minimal in the early stages of the disease. Examination of the sacroiliac joints and the spine (including the neck), measurement of chest expansion and range of motion of the hip and shoulder joints, and a search for signs of enthesitis are critical in making an early diagnosis of AS.[1–7] Important physical findings due to enthesitis that are present in many patients but are often overlooked include tenderness over vertebral spinal processes, iliac crest, anterior chest wall, calcaneus (plantar fasciitis and/or Achilles tendinitis), ischial tuberosities, greater trochanters, and sometimes tibial tubercles.

Tenderness may be noted over the sacroiliac joints, spinal processes, and other bony prominences. Direct pressure over the sacroiliac joint often, but not always, elicits pain if there is active sacroiliitis. Pain in the sacroiliac joint area may be elicited in some patients on sacroiliac stress testing by using maneuvers such as the FABERE test (hip Flexion, Abduction, External Rotation, and Extension). Sometimes sacroiliac pain may be elicited by pressure over the anterior superior iliac spines and on compressing the two iliac bones toward each other or forcing them away from each other (Fig. 6.1). Hyperextension of the lumbar spine or hyperextension of one hip joint while applying counterpressure on the iliac crest by the other hand, with the patient lying supine, can also be painful.

Tenderness and stiffness of the paraspinal muscles often accompany the inflammation of the axial skeleton, and the initial loss of spinal mobility is usually due to pain and muscle spasm rather than bony ankylosis. Therefore, marked improvement in spinal mobility can occur after treatment with NSAIDs and intensive physical therapy at an early stage of the disease.

The disease course and outcomes are quite variable in early stages, but generally a predictable pattern emerges within the first 10 years of disease. With longer disease duration and disease progression, there is a gradual loss of mobility of the lumbar spine. The entire spine becomes increasingly stiff, with loss of spinal mobility in all planes (Table 6.1). The patient loses normal posture after many years of disease progression; there is flattening of the lumbar spine and gradual development of accentuated dorsal (thoracic) spinal kyphosis.[1] The inflammatory process can extend to involve the cervical spine, and assessment of its range of motion, particularly lateral flexion, axial rotation, and hyperextension, should not be neglected. Temporomandibular joint pain and local tenderness occur in about 10% of patients, sometimes resulting in decreased range of motion of this joint.

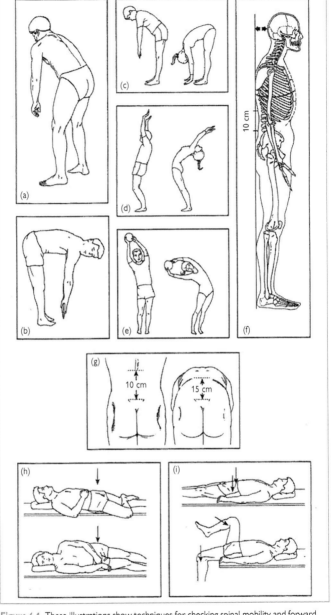

Figure 6.1 These illustrations show techniques for checking spinal mobility and forward stooping of the neck (also see Table 6.1), and for indirect compression of sacroiliac joints to elicit clinical evidence of sacroiliitis. A booklet providing further details has been published by Ankylosing Spondylitis International Federation (www.spondylitis-international.org). Reprinted with permission from Khan MA. *Ankylosing Spondylitis: The Facts*. Oxford: Oxford University Press; 2002.

Table 6.1 Measures of spinal mobility in AS

Measure*	Description
Cervical rotation	• Measure the angle of the cervical rotation using a goniometer.
	• Another method is to use a measuring tape to measure the distance between the tip of the nose and the acromioclavicular joint at baseline (when the neck is in neutral position) and on maximal ipsilateral rotation. A smaller difference indicates more restricted cervical rotation. The difference between these two positions measures the rotation and is measured separately for right/left and left/right rotations.
Fingertip-to-floor distance	• Distance between the tip of the right middle finger and the floor following maximal lumbar flexion, while maintaining full extension of the knees, measured ideally with a rigid tape measure. A smaller distance indicates greater movement.
Lumbar lateral flexion	• Distance between the tip of the ipsilateral middle finger and the floor following maximal lateral lumbar flexion, while maintaining heel contact with the floor, full extension of the knees, and without rotation of the trunk. This can be better achieved if the patient stands with the back against a wall. It is measured ideally with a rigid tape measure. A smaller distance indicates greater movement.
	• Domjan method (modified): A mark is made on the skin of one leg at the tip of the ipsilateral middle finger on maximal lateral lumbar flexion to that side, and another mark is placed on the same leg at the fingertip on maximal lateral lumbar flexion to the contralateral side. The distance between those two marks reflects lateral flexion of the lumbar spine.
Modified Schober's index	• Distance between two marks placed 10 cm apart on the lumbar spine in the midline, with the patient standing upright; the lower mark is at the level of the dimples of Venus or the posterior superior iliac spines. The distance between these two marks is measured again while the patient is maximally forward-flexing the spine, with the knees fully extended. Normally there is an increase of at least 5 cm (i.e., the distance between the two marks reaches 15 cm). An increase of <4 cm indicates decreased mobility of the lumbar spine.
Tragus-to-wall distance	• When the subject is standing erect with heels and buttocks against the wall (to prevent pivoting), knees fully extended and chin drawn in to keep a horizontal gaze, horizontal distance is measured with a rigid tape measure between the wall and the tragus of the right ear. A larger distance indicates worse forward stooping of the neck.
Occipital-to-wall distance	• When the subject is standing erect with heels and buttocks against the wall (to prevent pivoting), knees fully extended and chin drawn in to keep a horizontal gaze, horizontal distance is measured between the wall and the posterior convexity of the occiput. Subjects with normal posture show no gap. A larger distance indicates worse forward stooping of the neck.

* All measurements should be recorded after having the patient practice once.

Adapted from Haywood KL, Garratt AM, Jordan K, Dziedzic K, Dawes PT. Spinal mobility in ankylosing spondylitis: reliability, validity and responsiveness. *Rheumatology (Oxford)*. 2004;43:750–757.

Involvement of the costovertebral and costotransverse joints results in restricted chest expansion. A chest expansion of less than 2.5 cm at the xiphisternum level (or below the breasts in females) is abnormal (unless there is another reason for it, such as emphysema or scoliosis) and should raise the possibility of AS, especially in young patients with a history of chronic low back pain.

Although spinal ankylosis develops at a variable rate and pattern, the typical spinal deformities of AS usually evolve after 10 or more years. However, the disease occasionally remains confined to one part of the spine. Involvement of the cervical spine, usually one of the last musculoskeletal manifestations, results in progressive limitation of neck motion with a decreased ability to turn or extend the neck fully and a gradual development of forward stooping of the neck after many years.

Involvement of hip and shoulder joints

The hip and shoulder joints, the so-called girdle joints, are affected in at least one-third of AS patients. Hip joint involvement is usually bilateral and insidious (gradual) in onset; the pain is usually felt in the groin, although some patients feel it in the knee or the front of the thigh on the same side. There is a gradual destruction and thinning of the joint cartilage that cushions the bones of these joints, and it is accompanied by gradual limitation of joint motion.[1,2]

The reported frequency of hip joint involvement varies from 25% to 50%. It is more common when the disease starts at an earlier age. Some degree of contracture of the hip joints is not uncommon at later stages of the disease, giving rise to a characteristic rigid gait, with the patient keeping the knees bent a little in an attempt to maintain an erect posture. Shoulder joint involvement is generally mild. Involvement of the hip joints in a patient with a rigid spine, including the neck, is potentially more crippling and can lead to greater disability, but total hip joint replacement can minimize those limitations.

Involvement of peripheral joints other than the hips and shoulders is uncommon in "primary" AS. Such involvement is rarely persistent or destructive and tends to resolve without any residual joint deformity. Inflammation of the temporomandibular joint occurs in about 10% of cases; it causes pain, tenderness, or some limitation in fully opening the mouth.

Involvement of musculoskeletal structures other than entheses and joints

Spondylitis can also affect structures adjacent to the joints, such as tendons and bursae. Inflammation of these structures results in tendinitis and bursitis. There may be wasting and weakness of thigh and buttock muscles due to their lack of use in some patients, especially with advanced hip joint involvement.

AS in men and women

There has been in the past a greater degree of underdiagnosis of AS among women because the disease was wrongly considered to be much more common in men. For example, only 10% of the patients diagnosed around 1960 in Germany were females, but this percentage has increased in the subsequent decades to reach 46% among those diagnosed since 1990.[8] Women tend to have a milder disease course or atypical presentation and therefore may not be as easily diagnosed as men.[8] There is also a significantly longer delay in diagnosis among women. However, this delay in diagnosis is also getting shorter. The average age at onset of AS does not differ significantly among men and women. In some female patients, neck and peripheral joint involvement may be the main manifestation, and some may have symptoms that resemble "fibrositis" (fibromyalgia) or early rheumatoid arthritis.[1,9]

Spine fusion (ankylosis) may progress more slowly in women than in men. Functional outcome, as analyzed by studying activities of daily living, is similar in male and female patients. However, when it comes to pain and the need for drug therapy, female patients tend to be worse off than men with AS. It is possible that the slower and relatively incomplete progression of spinal fusion in female patients takes a longer time for a decrease of pain to occur as a consequence of complete spinal ankylosis.

AS in older patients

It is rare for AS to begin after the age of 45. However, there are many patients with AS whose disease is diagnosed at an older age, in part because they may have had minimal symptoms over the years. Some of them may present with back pain due to osteoporosis-related microfractures rather than due to inflammation. Treatment with simple, preferably non-narcotic analgesics may be safer than the use of NSAIDs in some of these patients, especially if they have stomach ulcers or underlying risk factors for ulcer disease, such as diabetes or cigarette smoking.

References

1. Khan MA. Ankylosing spondylitis: clinical features. In Hochberg M, Silman A, Smolen J, Weinblatt M, Weisman M, eds. *Rheumatology*, 3rd ed. London: Mosby: A Division of Harcourt Health Sciences Ltd., 2003:1161–1181.

2. Khan MA. Update on spondyloarthropathies. *Ann Intern Med.* 2002;136:896–907.

3. Khan MA. Spondyloarthropathies. In Hunder G, ed. *Atlas of Rheumatology*, 4th ed. Philadelphia: Current Medicine; 2005:151–180.

4. Rudwaleit M, Khan MA, Sieper J. How to diagnose axial SpA early. *Ann Rheum Dis.* 2004;63:535–543.

5. Khan MA, van der Linden SM, Kushner I, Valkenburg HA, Cats A. Spondylitic disease without radiological evidence of sacroiliitis in relatives of HLA-B27(+) patients. *Arthritis Rheum.* 1985;28:40–43.

6. Rudwaleit M, Khan MA, Sieper J. The challenge of diagnosis and classification in early ankylosing spondylitis: do we need new criteria? *Arthritis Rheum.* 2005;52:1000–1008.

7. Haywood KL, Garratt AM, Jordan K, Dziedzic K, Dawes PT. Spinal mobility in ankylosing spondylitis: reliability, validity and responsiveness. *Rheumatology (Oxford).* 2004;43:750–757.

8. Feldtkeller E, Khan MA, van der Linden S, van der Heijde D, Braun J. Age at disease onset and diagnosis delay in HLA-B27 negative vs. positive patients with ankylosing spondylitis. *Rheumatol Int.* 2003;23:61–66.

9. Lee W, Reveille JD, Weisman MH. Women with ankylosing spondylitis: a review. *Arthritis Rheum.* 2008;59(3):449–454.

Chapter 7

Diagnosis

Reliable early diagnosis of AS can be achieved even when, as in cases of axial undifferentiated disease, the conventional radiographic changes are absent.[1–6]

Why do we need an early diagnosis?

- To minimize or remove diagnostic uncertainty
- To initiate appropriate treatment early (e.g., NSAIDs, physical therapy, TNF-blocking agents)
- Because the burden of disease is substantial even in early disease (both in early AS and in undifferentiated axial SpA/preradiographic phase)
- Because TNF blockers work better in early stages of the disease (when inflammation is greater than destruction) than in late stages

As in other diseases where the etiology is not clearly defined, the diagnosis of AS is based primarily on the history and physical examination and is confirmed by radiographic examination.[1–8] A thorough clinical history and physical examination, particularly of the musculoskeletal system, are needed. Certain clinical features in the patient's history and physical examination raise the index of suspicion, and probably the best nonclinical indicator of the disease presence is finding radiographic evidence of sacroiliitis.

However, the status of the sacroiliac joints on routine pelvic radiographs is not always easy to interpret in the early phase of the disease, especially in adolescents.[8,9] Scintigraphy of the sacroiliac joints is at best of limited value for the diagnosis of established AS as well as the early diagnosis of probable or suspected sacroiliitis.[10,11] The diagnosis of AS is often missed or markedly delayed, especially in a primary care setting. A physician who is not fully aware of the various clinical presentations of AS might overlook this diagnosis when a teenager or a young adult presents with chronic back pain, even though this is a typical presentation. One of the reasons is that back pain is very prevalent in the general population, and AS or other related SpA are not its most common cause. Moreover, AS, like most other rheumatologic diseases, does not have a gold standard test that would make its diagnosis easy. Instead, the correct diagnosis depends largely on a constellation of clinical symptoms and signs in addition to radiographic findings.

Another challenge to an early diagnosis is that the disease starts insidiously, and symptoms can often be mild and nonspecific during the early stage of the disease. The progression of the disease is sometimes slow and minimally symptomatic. Furthermore, some patients may be pain free for long periods. There is also significant overlap in the clinical features of AS with the related SpA, especially during the early stages. Many cases of AS will be missed unless the physician has ample clinical experience and a high index of suspicion.

Active inflammation of the sacroiliac joints and spine is a common, early, and characteristic feature of AS and is present long before the appearance of unequivocal sacroiliitis or spondylitis on conventional radiography. Therefore, early diagnosis of AS is often challenging, but the absence of radiographic sacroiliitis during the early years of disease should not be used to rule out the diagnosis,[12] especially when the presence of inflammation can be detected by other, more costly, computer-generated imaging modalities, such as magnetic resonance imaging (MRI).[13–15] This use of MRI, especially the new technique of whole-body MRI, can detect the inflammatory response at an early stage (see Figs. 4.1 and 5.1).[15–17]

Sacroiliac plane radiographs are less reliable in detecting sacroiliitis in children and adolescents, and these patients may require MRI using STIR and other fat-suppression techniques that can demonstrate the inflammatory response associated with sacroiliitis and other sites of enthesitis without ionizing radiation. With the STIR technique, there is usually no need for gadolinium enhancement.[15] The inflammatory reaction involves not only the adjacent soft tissues but also the underlying bone marrow, and it sometimes extends a considerable distance away from the involved enthesis insertion (see Figs. 4.1 and 5.1). MRI is also very useful in detecting and evaluating complications of fractures or pseudarthrosis, as well as changes in the dura mater, soft tissue, and spinal ligaments.

During the past five decades there have been many attempts to establish clinical diagnostic criteria for AS. To date, there are no validated diagnostic criteria for AS and related SpA; all we have are the classification (not diagnostic) criteria (which are listed in Chapter 2). It is inappropriate for the clinicians to use classification criteria to establish the diagnosis because they are designed to be highly specific for the purpose of clinical studies to ensure that all the patients enrolled in a study have a firm diagnosis and that they are homogeneous. The classification criteria are therefore not sensitive enough to be used to establish the diagnosis in a clinical setting.

An early diagnosis has become increasingly important because effective therapies in the form of TNF antagonists have become available that are even more effective if used in early stages of the disease. Therefore, new strategies are being developed that will assist in making an early diagnosis and will also help primary care physicians in screening for these patients so that they can be referred to a rheumatologist when the disease is still in its early stages.[6,18] Studies are ongoing to develop diagnostic criteria for early AS using MRI (STIR technique without gadolinium enhancement), which has proven useful in detecting inflammation in the sacroiliac joints and spine in adults as well as in children.

In the meantime, to optimize the diagnostic accuracy of early or pre-radiographic AS (axial undifferentiated SpA), it is crucial to use a comprehensive approach and to have a deep understanding of the disease and its clinical picture. The clinician should gather a complete history, paying close attention to all the elements of this systemic disease, and should also use laboratory testing and imaging judiciously.[6,18,19]

A single clinical feature is not sufficient to make the diagnosis: the more features present that are typical of the disease, the higher the diagnostic probability. In the typical chronic low back pain population presenting to a primary care physician, back pain that meets the criteria for inflammatory back pain (see Tables 2.3 and 5.2) increases the probability of AS or axial SpA by a factor of 3, rising from less than 5% at baseline to more than 14%. In addition, if the patient has three or more of the additional clinical features listed in Table 7.1, the probability of disease presence can reach or exceed a comfort zone of diagnosis (>90% probability). In this case the diagnosis of axial undifferentiated spondylitis (or pre-radiographic AS) can be made in the absence of radiographic evidence of sacroiliitis, because the diagnosis (classification) of definite AS requires radiographic evidence of sacroiliitis.

Referral parameters have been developed that are easy for doctors in primary care to apply to patients presenting with possible AS; these could contribute to earlier diagnosis.[20,21] The proposed referral parameters have proven useful in Germany when applied in primary care (orthopedists and primary care doctors) to identify AS/pre-radiographic axial SpA in young to middle-aged patients with chronic low back pain.[21] Orthopedists and primary care doctors were asked to refer patients with (1) chronic low back pain (duration >3 months) and (2) onset of back pain before 45 years of age to a specialist rheumatology outpatient clinic for further diagnostic investigation if at least one of the following screening parameters was

Table 7.1 Diagnostic value of some clinical features of AS

Feature	Sensitivity (%)	Specificity (%)	(+)LR	(−)LR
Inflammatory-type back pain	75	76	3.1	0.33
Heel pain (enthesitis)	37	89	3.4	0.71
Peripheral arthritis	40	90	4.0	0.67
Dactylitis	18	96	4.5	0.85
Iritis/acute anterior uveitis	22	97	7.3	0.80
Positive family history (for AS, reactive or psoriatic arthritis, or uveitis)	32	95	6.4	0.72
Psoriasis	10	96	4.0	0.94
Inflammatory bowel disease	4	99	4.0	0.97
Good response to NSAIDs	77	85	5.1	0.27
Increased acute phase reactants (ESR/CRP)	50	80	2.5	0.63
HLA-B27 in whites*	90	90	9.0	0.11
Sacroiliitis revealed by MRI (STIR)	90	90	9.0	0.11

(+)LR, positive likelihood ratio; (−)LR, negative likelihood ratio; * patients of Northern European extraction suffering from primary AS. From Rudwaleit M, van der Heijde D, Khan MA, Braun J, Sieper J. How to diagnose axial spondyloarthropathy early. *Ann Rheum Dis.* 2004;63:535–543.

also present: (1) inflammatory back pain, (2) positive HLA- B27, and/or (3) sacroiliitis detected by imaging.

Laboratory findings

There are no specific laboratory markers that support the diagnosis of AS. Acute phase reactants such as elevated C-reactive protein (CRP) and erythrocyte sedimentation rate (ESR) are often used as part of the laboratory workup of inflammatory rheumatic diseases. Other acute-phase responses include elevated ferritin, mild thrombocytosis, and low albumin. The clinical use of ESR and CRP is limited, however, for diagnosing AS or related SpA because of their suboptimal sensitivity and specificity.[1–4] A normal ESR and CRP do not exclude the presence of clinically active AS. Although these tests usually correlate better with RA and polymyalgia rheumatica, they have less precise correlation with disease activity in AS. Elevated ESR and CRP are more commonly found in AS patients with peripheral arthritis than in those with only axial disease. Some may show anemia of chronic disease or high serum IgA levels, although studies seeking IgA antibodies to a variety of organisms have not been helpful. Testing for stool occult blood may be of value for inflammatory bowel disease. There is no association with rheumatoid factor and antinuclear antibody tests, and synovial fluid analysis and synovial biopsy are nonspecific.

When reactive arthritis is suspected on clinical grounds, bacterial studies (e.g., synovial fluid and throat cultures and tests for urogenital and enteric infection) might provide helpful information, although they may not be necessary for making the diagnosis.[22] Tests based on chlamydial lipopolysaccharide have a high sensitivity but cannot differentiate between *Chlamydia trachomatis* and *Chlamydia pneumoniae* infections. Use of *C. trachomatis*–specific peptides from the major outer membrane protein (MOMP) can help differentiate between the chlamydial species or even serovars. It is unusual, especially in the postenteritic form of ReA, to isolate a microbial trigger after ReA has developed. Stool cultures are needed for detecting enteric infection by disease-triggering bacteria, but a negative result does not exclude the diagnosis of ReA or its enteric trigger when there is a history of diarrhea. It is not uncommon for the stool cultures to become negative by the time patients seek medical help because of arthritis.

In acute *Yersinia*-induced ReA, IgG plus IgA antibodies can be detected in almost all patients, and IgA antibodies can still be detectable in more than 80% after a year. However, DNA of these bacteria is only rarely detected inside the joint, and it has been suggested that rather mucosa and lymph nodes might serve as a reservoir for *Yersinia* and *Salmonella*. Therefore, a *Salmonella*- or *Yersinia*-specific polymerase chain reaction (PCR) for joint material does not currently play a clinically helpful role in the diagnosis of ReA.[22] The use of serology for the diagnosis of infections with *C. trachomatis* is hampered by the relatively high prevalence of positive antibody titers among controls and by a possible cross-reactivity with antibodies directed against *C. pneumoniae*.[22] Antibody titers should be elevated at least 2 standard deviations above that of the control population. Antibodies of the IgG subclass alone do not reflect a recent infection well enough because they can remain elevated for months after an infection, whereas IgM and IgA antibodies reflect an acute or persistent infection.[22] However, these antibodies can also be positive in a control population with a high infection rate. resulting in a reduced specificity of this test. HIV testing should be considered in high-risk patients and in patients with recent onset of florid psoriasis or ReA.

HLA-B27 test

HLA-B27 is a normal gene; its prevalence in the general population and the strength of its association with AS and related SpA markedly differ among the various ethnic and racial groups worldwide (Tables 7.2 and 7.3). Moreover, many of these patients can lack this gene, especially in certain populations. For example, HLA-B27 is present in only 3% of

Table 7.2 Association of HLA-B27 and AS and related SpA in whites of northern European extraction

Disease	Approximate HLA-B27 Prevalence (%)
Ankylosing spondylitis (primary AS)	85 to 95
Reactive arthritis	40 to 80
Juvenile spondyloarthropathy	≈70
Enteropathic spondylitis	35 to 75
Psoriatic spondylitis	40 to 50
Undifferentiated spondyloarthropathy	≈70
Acute anterior uveitis (acute iritis)	≈50
Aortic incompetence with heart block	≈80
General healthy population	≈8

The association of HLA-B27 with AS and related SpA is much weaker in some racial/ethnic groups; for example, only about 50% of African American patients with primary AS possess HLA-B27.[23]

Table 7.3 Marked differences in the worldwide general prevalence of HLA-B27 in various population groups

Population groups	HLA-B27 freqeuncy (%)
Caucasoid population groups	
Ugro-Finnish	12 to 18
Northern Scandinavians	10 to 16
Slavic populations	7 to 14
Western Europeans	6 to 9
Southern Europeans	2 to 6
Sardinians	5
Basques	9 to 14
Gypies(Spain)	16 to 18
Turks	7 to 14

49

Table 7.3 continued

Population groups	HLA-B27 freqeuncy (%)
Arabs*, Jews, Armenians & Iranian	3 to 5
Pakistanis	6 to 8
Indians (Asian)	2 to 6
Native American Populations divided by linguistic groups	
Eskimo-Aleut	25 to 40
Na-Dane (Haida, Tlingit, Dogrib, Navajo)	20 to 40
Amerind	
North American	7 to 26
Mexicans Mestizo	3 to 6
Central American	4 to 20
South American	0
North and South Asiatic linguistic populations groups	
Chukchic	19 to 40
Uralic	8 to 24
Altaic	
Siberians	6 to 19
Japanese	<1
Ainu (Native Japanese)	4
Koreans	3 to 8
Mongolians	3 to 9
Uygurs, Kazakhs, Turkic, Uzbek	3 to 8
Sino-Tibetan	
Chinese	2 to 9
Tibetans	12
Other Asiatic populations groups	
Indonesians	5 to 12
Malaysians and Filipinos	4 to 5
Micronesians (Nauru, Guam)	2 to 5
Melanesians (Papua New Guinea, Fiji, etc.)	4 to 53
Polynesians	0 to 3
Australian Aboriginies	0
African populations groups	
North Africans	1 to 5
West Africans (Mali, Gambia & Senegal)	2 to 10
Pygmies	7 to 10
Bantu (Nigeria, Southern Africa)	0
San (Bushmen)	0

*Prevelance of B27 may be much lower (doser to 1%) in the United Arab Emirates and adjacent parts of Saudi Arabia, and among Lebanese Maronite Christion Arabs.

The numbers are rounded off for simplicity and indicate percentage prevalence in the general population.

the African American general population and only about 50% of patients with AS.[23,24]

HLA-B27 is a relatively inexpensive test and it does not need to be repeated (unless for technical/laboratory error). However, it cannot be thought of as a routine, diagnostic, confirmatory, or screening test for AS in patients presenting with back pain or arthritis. As a rule, if the history and physical examination findings suggest AS but the radiographic findings do not permit this diagnosis to be made, this test may allow the presumptive diagnosis of AS to be accepted or rejected with less uncertainty. In patients with back pain or arthritis in whom the clinical history and physical examination findings do not suggest AS, testing for HLA-B27 will be inappropriate because a positive result would still not permit the diagnosis of AS to be made.[1,3,24,25]

The value of this test in diagnosing AS depends on the individual probability of the disease when the test is ordered and the patient's ethnicity and race. The test is most useful if the pretest probability is approximately 50% (toss-up) or in the range of 30% to 70%, if sacroiliac radiography findings are normal or equivocal, and if MRI is not available or affordable.[24,25]

A negative HLA-B27 test in African Americans is clinically not very helpful in lowering the pretest probability of AS, but a positive test is more helpful as an aid to diagnosis among them (positive likelihood ratio ≈17) than in whites (positive likelihood ratio ≈10).[1,24,25] The test is very useful in Japanese patients with suspected AS because of its strong association with AS (≈80%) and a less than 1% prevalence of HLA-B27 in the general Japanese population (positive likelihood ratio >100).

As explained earlier, back pain and stiffness due to AS can often precede unequivocal radiographic signs of sacroiliitis by several years. Therefore, the status of the sacroiliac joints on a pelvic radiograph are not always easy to interpret in the early phase of the disease, particularly in adolescents, although MRI, a costly technique, can help to detect early sacroiliitis in this clinical situation without causing any gonadal radiation.[15] Alternatively, an early diagnosis of AS or axial SpA can be made with much less uncertainty when a test for HLA-B27 is ordered in a toss-up situation (30% to 70% pretest probability of AS) and the result is positive. However, currently the diagnosis of AS depends heavily on the radiographic evidence of sacroiliitis, which is the best nonclinical indicator of the disease presence.

HLA-B27 typing may help ophthalmologists to better classify a patient presenting with acute uveitis and to refer HLA-B27-positive patients for rheumatology consultation, especially those with associated musculoskeletal symptoms, because up to 75% of them have or will develop AS or a related SpA.

Although HLA-B27 typing can define the population at higher risk of AS and related SpA, it is of very limited practical value for that purpose in the general population because no effective means of prevention is currently available, and most B27-positive individuals never develop AS or a related disease. The risk of development of AS or any type of SpA even among B27-positive first-degree relatives of a B27-positive patient with AS is only 20%; it is very much lower in the general public with B27.[24,25]

Imaging

Radiographic evidence of sacroiliitis is a characteristic feature of AS.[1,8] It usually is bilateral and symmetrical in primary AS and typically first involves the lower synovial part of the joint (Fig. 7.1). Obtaining an anteroposterior radiograph of the pelvis usually is sufficient to detect sacroiliitis in established disease (see Fig. 1.2A), but the results may be normal or equivocal early in the disease course. One should avoid ordering oblique views of the sacroiliac joints as they are difficult to obtain, are associated with significant radiation exposure, and do not provide much added information.

MRI using the STIR technique, without the need for gadolinium enhancement, may detect sacroiliitis and spondylitis long before these abnormalities become evident on plane radiography[15-17] and thus offer the clinician an opportunity for early diagnosis. The recently described whole-body MRI scan very nicely identifies the characteristic bone edema that results from osteitis/enthesitis at axial as well as peripheral sites, and it takes only 30 minutes to perform[13-17] (see Figs. 4.1 and 5.1). CT of the SI joints may also be helpful if MRI is not available or cannot be used, but it is associated with significant gonadal irradiation. Technetium-99m bone scanning is not very helpful for early detection of sacroiliitis, but it may be used to detect pseudarthrosis or fracture.

The earliest lesions in AS are usually detectable in the caudal part of the synovial segment of the sacroiliac joint by MRI; the joint capsule, enthesis, and subchondral bone are probably the earliest sites involved[15,17] (see Fig. 7.1). MRI also reveals that the lower thoracic and upper lumbar spine can

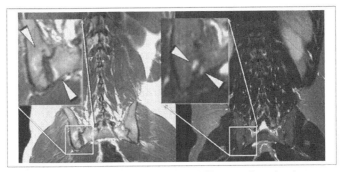

Figure 7.1 These coronal sections of whole-body MRI were performed on the same day in 25-year-old HLA-B27-positive identical twins with a highly concordant onset of spondyloarthropathy, sites of involvement, and disease course. (*Left*) This T1-weighted image from twin A shows chronic inflammatory changes of the right sacroiliac joint (erosion, sclerosing joint margins, and fatty replacement of subchondral bone marrow on both sides of the joint) 11 months after onset of right-sided buttock pain. (*Right*) This STIR sequence is from twin B, who had a few weeks of lumbar morning stiffness but no back or gluteal pain. Subtle acute inflammatory lesions are present in the distal (caudal) part of the right sacroiliac joint, on both the iliac and the sacral sides. The inset shows magnification of the involved sites. Reprinted, with permission from the *Journal of Rheumatology*, from Weber U, Pfirrmann CWA, Kissling RO, MacKenzie CR, Khan MA. Early spondyloarthritis in HLA-B27 positive monozygotic twin pair: a highly concordant onset, sites of involvement, and disease course. *J Rheumatol.* 2008;35(7):1464–1467.

become involved early with skip lesions, indicating that the spinal involvement in early AS does not always extend in an orderly fashion from the sacroiliac joint upward (see Figs. 4.1 and 5.1). The entheseal bone edema can be evident on MRI at entheses adjacent to synovial joints and at the bony attachment of the joint capsule (see Fig. 4.1), and also at sites devoid of synovium such as the plantar fascia.

In peripheral enthesitis, it is possible to visualize inflammatory processes in tendons and ligaments by high-frequency real-time ultrasonography. This is a relatively inexpensive method for assessing enthesitis, although it is operator dependent. It can demonstrate entheseal swelling, tendinitis, peritendinous soft tissue swelling, bursitis, and ligamentous and periosteal swelling. Enthesitis is associated with alterations of the normal fibrillar echo texture: the echogenicity of the enthesis is decreased due to inflammation and edema and possibly bone erosion or new bone formation at the insertion. The conventional radiographic features of enthesitis include soft tissue swelling, osteopenia and/or bony sclerosis at entheseal bone insertions, bone cortex irregularity at insertions and adjacent periostitis, as well as entheseal soft tissue calcification and new bone formation.

Entheseal structures have low water content and are therefore not well visualized on MRI; the adjacent soft tissue and bone changes ("bone edema" due to osteitis) are best seen. Dynamic (gadolinium-enhanced) MRI and the use of STIR and other fat-suppression techniques show that the inflammatory response associated with enthesitis may be extensive. It involves not only the adjacent soft tissues but also the underlying bone marrow, and it sometimes extends a considerable distance away from the enthesis insertion (see Figs. 4.1 and 5.1). Widespread inflammation in the spine as detected by MRI contributes to predicting a major clinical response (BASDAI 50 response) in active AS patients treated with anti-TNF agents.[26]

Spinal osteopenia, which is common, correlates with disease severity and duration. Measurements of bone density of the spine by dual-energy x-ray absorptiometry (DEXA) scan to detect osteoporosis may be less reliable than measurements at the femoral neck because of the presence of spinal syndesmophytes and ligamentous ossification. Peripheral DEXA scans may be used in patients who have had bilateral hip arthroplasty.

Radiographic findings in patients with spondylitis secondary to PsA or ReA may be asymmetrical, with skip lesions or nonmarginal, large, asymmetrical syndesmophytes, or both (see Fig. 1.2F). Conventional radiographs may also reveal soft tissue swelling or erosive changes in the peripheral joints of patients with PsA and ReA. Some of the classical findings of PsA include periostitis, bony ankylosis, and destructive "pencil-in-cup" deformities (a bone's distal head becomes pointed and the adjacent joint surface becomes cuplike because of erosions in the fingers and toes[3]). Periarticular osteopenia, often seen in RA, is generally not a feature in PsA.

Radiographic evidence of sacroiliitis, especially unilateral or asymmetrical, may also result from other causes—including infections (e.g., brucellosis

Table 7.4 Features differentiating DISH (ankylosing hyperostosis) from AS

Feature	Ankylosing hyperostosis	Ankylosing spondylitis
Usual age of onset (years)	>50	<40
Thoracolumbar kyphosis	±	++
Limitation of spinal mobility	±	++
Pain	±	++
Limitation of chest expansion	±	++
Radiographic features:		
Hyperostosis	++	+
Sacroiliac joint erosion	––	++
Sacroiliac joint (synovial) obliteration	±	++
Sacroiliac joint (ligamentous) obliteration	±	++
Apophyseal joint obliteration	––	++
Anterior longitudinal ligament ossification	++	±
Posterior longitudinal ligament ossification	+	?
Syndesmophytes	––	++
Enthesopathies (whiskerings) with erosions	––	++
Enthesopathies (whiskerings) without erosions	++	+

Reprinted, with permission from Lippincott, Williams and Wilkins, Inc., from Yagan R, Khan MA. Confusion of roentgenographic differential diagnosis of ankylosing hyperostosis (Forestier's disease) and ankylosing spondylitis. *Spine: State of the Art Reviews*. 1990;4:561–575.

and tuberculosis)—but the clinical presentation usually is sufficiently discernible from that of AS and related SpA. Osteitis condensans ilii (sclerosis of the iliac side of the sacroiliac joints without cortical erosions or joint space changes) also must be distinguished from sacroiliitis in women, especially those with history of multiple pregnancies.[27]

Ankylosing hyperostosis, also called Forestier disease or diffuse idiopathic skeletal hyperostosis (DISH), can cause excessive new bone formation along the spine and other sites (e.g., at entheses); this can result in a stiff spine that may be confused with AS, but it usually occurs in older patients.[3,28–30] It is characterized by a flowing ligamentous ossification, especially of the anterior longitudinal ligament, and the absence of typical sacroiliitis, although capsular ossification may diminish the clarity of the sacroiliac and facet joints on radiographic images (Table 7.4).

Another illness that can cause confusion is a rare disease of uncertain etiology that is known by many different names but is most commonly called SAPHO syndrome.[31,32] It is so named because of its salient features: Synovitis, Acne, Palmoplantar pustulosis, Hyperostosis, and aseptic Osteomyelitis. It causes aseptic bone necrosis at multiple sites, which can include the sacroiliac joints or the spine, with associated back pain. Other differential diagnoses include Paget's disease (of the pelvis and spine) and Scheuermann's disease. Spread of cancer to the pelvis and the spine, as well as some chronic spinal infections, can also present as back pain.[33,34]

Other causes of back pain

Pain in the back is very prevalent, probably second only to the common cold as a cause of discomfort and incapacity necessitating a visit to the primary care physician. It is the most common reason for temporary disability for persons under 45 years of age, and close to 80% of Americans will have a low back problem of some type at least once by age 50. The various causes of back pain can be broadly divided into the following categories:

- Local reasons in the vertebral column ("spondylogenic"), which could be traumatic, structural (e.g., osteoporosis), mechanical (e.g., disc degeneration, spondylolisthesis), inflammatory (e.g., ankylosing spondylitic), congenital, or metabolic, or the result of infection, cancer, or other bone lesions
- Nonspondylogenic causes (e.g., neurologic, vascular, or psychological, or referred from disease in the pelvis [gynecological] and abdomen)

By far the most common cause is mechanical deterioration of the spine, with its many forms and presentations. Clinical back pain related to disc degeneration increases with age and is accelerated by mechanical stress.

Over 85% of a child's disc in its central part is composed of water, and there is a slow but steady decrease with aging, down to about 60% by the age of 80 years. These changes result in a diminished volume of the disc, leading to narrowing of the disc space, with resultant buckling of the surrounding ligaments (annulus fibrosus and spinal ligaments) and bony spur formation (osteophytes) at the edges of the spinal vertebral bodies.

There are many other causes of back pain reviewed elsewhere in excellent publications.[33,34] Some of these causes include spinal osteoporosis (with or without compression fractures) and osteomalacia. Osteomalacia results from dietary deficiency of vitamin D and lack of adequate skin exposure to sunlight, or from chronic kidney failure. It can cause back pain and can be mistaken for AS and related SpAs, or it can co-occur with these diseases.

References

1. Khan MA. Ankylosing spondylitis: clinical features. In Hochberg M, Silman A, Smolen J, Weinblatt M, Weisman M, eds. *Rheumatology*, 3rd ed. London: Mosby: A Division of Harcourt Health Sciences Ltd.; 2003:1161–1181.

2. Khan MA. Update on spondyloarthropathies. *Ann Intern Med*. 2002; 136:896–907.

3. Khan MA. Spondyloarthropathies. In Hunder G, ed. *Atlas of Rheumatology*, 4th ed. Philadelphia: Current Medicine; 2005:151–180.

4. Rudwaleit M, Khan MA, Sieper J. How to diagnose axial SpA early. *Ann Rheum Dis*. 2004;63:535–543.

5. Khan MA, van der Linden SM, Kushner I, Valkenburg, HA, Cats A. Spondylitic disease without radiological evidence of sacroiliitis in relatives of HLA-B27(+) patients. *Arthritis Rheum*. 1985;28:40–43.

6. Rudwaleit M, Khan MA, Sieper J. The challenge of diagnosis and classification in early ankylosing spondylitis: do we need new criteria? *Arthritis Rheum.* 2005;52:1000–1008.

7. Haywood KL, Garratt AM, Jordan K, Dziedzic K, Dawes PT. Spinal mobility in ankylosing spondylitis: reliability, validity and responsiveness. *Rheumatology (Oxford).* 2004;43:750–757.

8. Tuite MJ. Sacroiliac joint imaging. *Semin Musculoskelet Radiol.* 2008;12(1):72–82.

9. van Tubergen A, Heuft-Dorenbosch L, Schulpen G, et al. Radiographic assessment of sacroiliitis by radiologists and rheumatologists: does training improve quality? *Ann Rheum Dis.* 2003;62(6):519–525.

10. Miron SD, Khan MA, Wiesen E, Kushner I, Bellon EM. The value of quantitative sacroiliac scintigraphy in detection of sacroiliitis. *Clin Rheumatol.* 1983;2:407–414.

11. Song IH, Carrasco-Fernández J, Rudwaleit M, Sieper J. The diagnostic value of scintigraphy in assessing sacroiliitis in ankylosing spondylitis—a systematic literature research. *Ann Rheum Dis.* 2008 Jan 29 [Epub ahead of print].

12. Khan MA, van der Linden SM, Kushner I, Valkenburg HA, Cats A. Spondylitic disease without radiological evidence of sacroiliitis in relatives of HLA-B27 positive patients. *Arthritis Rheum.* 1985;28:40–43.

13. Oostveen J, Prevo R, den Boer J, van de Laar M. Early detection of sacroiliitis on magnetic resonance imaging and subsequent development of sacroiliitis on plain radiography. A prospective, longitudinal study. *J Rheumatol.* 1999;26(9):1953–1958.

14. Hermann KG, Landewe RB, Braun J, van der Heijde DM. Magnetic resonance imaging of inflammatory lesions in the spine in ankylosing spondylitis clinical trials: is paramagnetic contrast medium necessary? *J Rheumatol.* 2005;32(10):2056–2060.

15. Weber U, Kissling JO, Hodler J. Advances in musculoskeletal imaging and their clinical utility in the early diagnosis of spondyloarthritis. *Curr Rheumatol Rep.* 2007;9(5):353–360.

16. Weber U, Pfirrmann CWA, Khan MA. Ankylosing spondylitis: update on imaging and therapy. *Intl J Adv Rheumatol.* 2007;5:2–7.

17. Weber U, Pfirrmann CWA, Kissling RO, MacKenzie CR, Khan MA. Early spondyloarthritis in HLA-B27 positive monozygotic twin pair: a highly concordant onset, sites of involvement, and disease course. *J Rheumatol.* 2008;35(7):1464–1467.

18. Rudwaleit M, Metter A, Listing J, Sieper J, Braun J. Inflammatory back pain in ankylosing spondylitis: a reassessment of the clinical history for application as classification and diagnostic criteria. *Arthritis Rheum.* 2006;54(2):569–578.

19. Rudwaleit M, van der Heijde D, Khan MA, Braun J, Sieper J. How to diagnose axial spondyloarthropathy early. *Ann Rheum Dis.* 2004;63:535–543.

20. Song I-H, Sieper J, Rudwaleit M. Diagnosing early ankylosing spondylitis. *Curr Rheumatol Rep.* 2007;9(5):367–344.

21. Brandt HC, Spiller I, Song IH, Vahldiek JL, Rudwaleit M, Sieper J. Performance of referral recommendations in patients with chronic back pain and suspected axial spondyloarthritis. *Ann Rheum Dis.* 2007;66(11):1479–1484.

22. Khan MA, Sieper J. Reactive arthritis. In Koopman WJ, Moreland LW, eds. *Arthritis and Allied Conditions,* 15th ed. Philadelphia: Lippincott Williams & Wilkins; 2004:1335–1355.

23. Khan MA, Braun WE, Kushner I, Grecek DE, Muir WA, Steinberg AG. HLA B27 in ankylosing spondylitis: differences in frequency and relative risk in American Blacks and Caucasians. *J Rheumatol Suppl.* 1977;3:39–43.

24. Khan MA, Khan MK. Diagnostic value of HLA-B27 testing in ankylosing spondy-litis and Reiter's syndrome. *Ann Intern Med.* 1982;96:70–76.

25. Khan MA. How the B27 test can help in the diagnosis of spondyloarthropa-thies. In Calin A, ed. *Spondyloarthropathies.* New York: Grune & Stratton; 1984:323–337.

26. Rudwaleit M, Schwarzlose S, Hilgert ES, Listing J, Braun J, Sieper J. MRI in pre-dicting a major clinical response to anti-tumor necrosis factor treatment in ankylosing spondylitis. *Ann Rheum Dis.* 2008;67:1276–1281.

27. Olivieri I, Gemignani G, Camerini E, et al. Differential diagnosis between osteitis condensans ilii and sacroiliitis. *J Rheumatol.* 1990;17(11):1504–1512. Erratum in *J Rheumatol.* 1991;18(5):790.

28. Yagan R, Khan MA. Confusion of roentgenographic differential diagnosis of ankylosing hyperostosis (Forestier's disease) and ankylosing spondylitis. *Spine: State of the Art Reviews.* 1990;4(3):561–575.

29. Yagan R, Khan MA. Confusion of roentgenographic differential diagnosis between ankylosing hyperostosis (Forestier's disease) and ankylosing spondy-litis. *Clin Rheumatol.* 1983;2:285–292.

30. Olivieri I, D'Angelo S, Cutro MS, et al. Diffuse idiopathic skeletal hyperostosis may give the typical postural abnormalities of advanced ankylosing spondylitis. *Rheumatology (Oxford).* 2007;46(11):1709–1711.

31. Kahn M-F, Khan MA. SAPHO syndrome. *Ballieres Clin Rheumatol.* 1994;8:333–362.

32. Hayem G, Bouchaud-Chabot A, Benali K, et al. SAPHO syndrome: a long-term follow-up study of 120 cases. *Semin Arthritis Rheum.* 1999;29:159–171.

33. Diamond S, Borenstein D. Chronic low back pain in a working-age adult. *Best Pract Res Clin Rheumatol.* 2006;20(4):707–720.

34. Carragee EJ. Clinical practice. Persistent low back pain. *N Engl J Med.* 2005;352(18):1891–1898.

Chapter 8

Other manifestations and complications

Ocular manifestations

Acute anterior uveitis, also called acute iritis, is the most common extraarticular feature of AS, occurring in 25% to 40% of patients at some time in the course of their disease[1-4] (Fig. 8.1). It is an acute inflammation of the iris and ciliary body and is therefore also called acute iritis or iridocyclitis. It is typically unilateral, and the symptoms usually begin acutely and include pain, increased lacrimation, photophobia, and some blurring of vision. It has a tendency to recur, not infrequently in the contralateral eye.

The eye is inflamed, there is circumcorneal congestion, the pupil is small, and the iris is edematous and may appear slightly discolored compared to the contralateral side. There is copious exudate in the anterior chamber of the eye, which can be seen on slit-lamp examination. The inflammation is nongranulomatous—that is, the inflammatory cells adhering to the endothelial lining cells of the cornea form aggregates called keratitic precipitates, which are small, in contrast to what is usually seen in "granulomatous uveitis" of sarcoidosis and some other diseases.

The individual attack of acute uveitis usually subsides within a few weeks without any sequelae, but residual visual impairment may occur if treatment is inadequate or delayed. The pupil may become irregular if the iritis is not properly treated and the inflamed iris becomes attached posteriorly

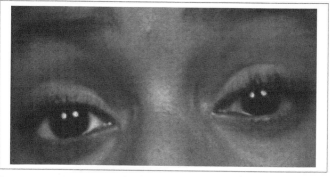

Figure 8.1 This photograph shows acute anterior uveitis of the left eye.
Source: Khan MA. Ankylosing spondylitis: clinical features. In Hochberg M, Silman A, Smolen J, Weinblatt M, Weisman M, eds. *Rheumatology*, 3rd ed. London: Mosby: A Division of Harcourt Health Sciences Ltd.; 2003:1161–1181. Reprinted with permission from Elsevier.

to the lens, causing posterior synechiae formation, or anteriorly to the cornea, causing anterior synechiae formation. Such complications can lead to secondary glaucoma and cataract in the long run. In a few cases, the posterior chamber also becomes inflamed, resulting in macular edema and further visual blurring.

The prevalence of uveitis varies with the type of SpA. On average 33% of AS patients and 25% of psoriatic arthritis patients have one or more episodes of uveitis, and this percentage increases with disease duration. It is significantly more common in HLA-B27-positive versus B27-negative patients, with an odds ratio of 4.2.[4,5] The uveitis is acute, anterior, and unilateral close to 90% of the time; recurrences occur in 50% of patients, and it rarely (8%) results in a reduction of visual acuity. One should rule out associated inflammatory bowel disease or psoriasis if the uveitis begins insidiously, lasts longer than 6 months, or is bilateral or involves the posterior uveal tract.

Occasionally uveitis is the presenting symptom that draws attention to the diagnosis of AS or related SpA. HLA-B27-positive acute anterior uveitis is the most common definable type of uveitis, representing about 15% of all kinds of uveitis.

Cardiac manifestations

Recent studies, particularly those using transesophageal echocardiography, suggest that cardiovascular involvement in patients with AS is more common than previously realized.[1–3,6] Inflammation at the aortic root (aortitis) causes intimal proliferation and adventitial scarring of the vasa vasorum. This can lead to fibrosis with hemodynamically unimportant consequences or a dilated aortic ring, thickened and shortened aortic valves with nodularities of the aortic cusps, and basal thickening of the anterior mitral leaflet and the adjacent ventricular septum, forming the characteristic "subaortic bump." This "bump" or thickened valvular cusps can be detected by transthoracic and transesophageal echocardiography in more than 30% of AS patients without any clinically apparent heart disease. Extension of the fibrotic process into the atrioventricular conduction bundle can cause heart block.

The risk for aortic insufficiency and cardiac conduction disturbances increases with the age of the patient, the duration of AS, the presence of HLA-B27, and peripheral joint involvement. For example, cardiac conduction disturbances occur in up to 3% of those with disease of 15 years' duration and up to 9% after 30 years. Complete heart block causing Stokes-Adams attacks may supervene in some patients, necessitating implantation of a cardiac pacemaker. The aortic regurgitation follows a chronic but relentless course to heart failure, usually over several years, necessitating valvular replacement. Sometimes acute aortic (and rarely even mitral) insufficiency with rapid deterioration of cardiac function occurs in relatively young patients with minimal spondylitis.

Occurrence of the cardiac syndrome of "lone aortic incompetence and pacemaker-requiring bradycardia" in men without spondyloarthropathy is an HLA-B27-associated inflammatory condition. Among 91 patients with the combination of heart block and aortic insufficiency, 88% had HLA-B27, and only about 20% of them had AS or a related SpA. There is no association between HLA-B27 and lone aortic incompetence in the absence of complete heart block or SpA. However, HLA-B27 was found to be more common (17%) among 83 patients with isolated complete heart block (without any clinical or radiographic evidence of associated SpA) than in normal controls (6%).

Pulmonary manifestations

Rigidity of the chest wall in patients with AS results in inability to expand the chest fully on inspiration and can result in mild restrictive lung function impairment.[1–3,7,8] However, this does not usually result in ventilatory insufficiency because of increased diaphragmatic contribution. Pleuropulmonary involvement can occur as a rare (1% to 2% of patients) and late extraskeletal manifestation in the form of a slowly progressive and usually bilateral apical pulmonary fibrosis that appears as linear or patchy opacities on chest radiographs and eventually become cystic. These cavitations may mimic tuberculosis lesions and may become colonized by *Aspergillus* species with the formation of mycetoma. The patient may complain of cough, increasing dyspnea, and occasionally hemoptysis.

Newer imaging modalities, such as thin-section high-resolution CT, indicate that there is general underappreciation of the pulmonary parenchymal involvement in AS.[7,8] These abnormalities are usually subtle and subclinical, mostly comprising thickening of the interlobular septa, mild bronchial wall or pleural thickening, pleuropulmonary irregularities, and linear septal thickening. They do not correlate with functional and clinical impairment.

Gastrointestinal manifestations

Apart from the well-known association of chronic inflammatory bowel diseases with AS, clinically silent (asymptomatic) enteric mucosal inflammatory lesions, both macroscopic and microscopic, have been detected in the terminal ileum and proximal colon on ileocolonoscopic studies in more than 50% of AS patients with no gastrointestinal symptoms.[9–11] This supports the existence of a pathogenic link between gut inflammation and AS, and it is independent of HLA-B27. Follow-up studies of such patients indicate that 6% of them will develop inflammatory bowel disease, and among those with histologically "chronic" inflammatory gut lesions 15% to 25% will develop clinically obvious Crohn's disease, suggesting that the latter group of patients had initially a subclinical form of Crohn's disease when they presented with arthritis.

The appearance of SpA in patients with inflammatory bowel disease is not related to the extent of the bowel disease. Symptomatic or asymptomatic sacroiliitis is related to the disease duration. Asymptomatic sacroiliitis is a common manifestation of inflammatory bowel disease, occurring in almost 20% of the patients. In addition, close to 40% of the patients have joint symptoms, and among them 10% can be classified as having AS, and an additional 80% meet the criteria for other forms of SpA.

Osteoporosis

Spinal osteoporosis is commonly observed, especially in patients with severe AS of long duration. It is partly a result of ankylosis and lack of mobility but may also be related to a mineralization defect in AS.[12,13] A marked reduction in bone mineral density of the lumbar spine and femoral neck has been reported on dual energy x-ray absorptiometry (DEXA) measurement in a group of young patients with early AS. It may result from proinflammatory cytokines and contributes to vertebral compression fractures and progressive spinal deformity in some patients. Bone biopsies and assessment of biochemical markers of bone metabolism have shown that both diminished bone formation and enhanced bone resorption are involved. One should also look for concomitant deficiency of vitamin D.

Spondylodiscitis and spinal fractures

An aseptic spondylodiscitis, mostly in the midthoracic spine, and usually asymptomatic and without any physical trauma, can occur and is relatively more common in the patients whose spondylitis also involves the cervical spine.[12–15] There is also an increased prevalence of vertebral compression fractures, discovertebral destructive lesions (so-called Andersson lesions), and spinal fractures.

The ankylosed spine breaks like a long bone, and the fracture line is usually transverse; it is more often transdiscal (across syndesmophytes) than transvertebral. The rigid osteoporotic spine is unduly susceptible to fracture even after relatively minor trauma, including events that may not be recalled by the patient. One should exclude the possibility of spinal fracture in any patient with advanced AS who complains of new onset of neck or back pain, even in the absence of a definite trauma. The cervical spine, usually at the C5–6 or C6–7 level, is the most common site of fracture; quadriplegia can result, especially if associated with dislocation, and this is a very serious complication with a high morbidity and mortality. Neurologic deficits are often subtle on initial presentation, resulting in missed diagnosis because of a low index of suspicion and poor visualization of lower cervical fractures on conventional radiography.

Before any imaging studies, the ankylosed and forwardly stooped cervical spine in a patient with cervicothoracic kyphosis must be immobilized in the patient's usual alignment, because excessive extension into "normal" posture during conventional immobilization or for radiologic procedures can result in neurologic deficits and may make a stable fracture unstable. Such patients should carry Medical Alert cards (see Table 13.1) that should identify the degree of forward stooping of the neck and the precautions that need to be instituted by emergency services for their care if they have an accident.

Sometimes an undiagnosed or improperly treated fracture results in spondylodiscitis and pseudarthrosis and can lead to severe kyphotic deformities.[12–15] The diagnosis of these fractures may be difficult in a "bamboo spine," and focal spinal abnormalities on bone scans can be a clue to the presence of fracture or pseudarthrosis. MRI and CT are important in detecting and evaluating complications of fractures or pseudarthrosis, as well as changes in the dura mater, soft tissue, and longitudinal ligaments.

Atlantoaxial subluxation

Erosions of the odontoid process and the transverse ligament can result in spontaneous atlantoaxial subluxation, usually anteriorly. It can present as occipital pain, with or without signs of spinal cord compression, and is more common in patients with peripheral joint involvement.[3,12,15] It generally occurs in the later stages of the disease, although it can be an early manifestation.[16] Vertical (upward migration of the odontoid process into the brain stem [platybasia]), rotatory, posterior atlantoaxial, or subaxial subluxations and fracture of the odontoid process have been reported rarely.

Neurologic manifestations

Neurologic involvement may occur in patients with AS and is related most often to fracture-dislocation of the spine, cauda equina syndrome, or atlantoaxial subluxation.[3,12,15] A slowly progressive cauda equina syndrome is a rare but significant complication of long-standing AS; it results from fibrous entrapment and scarring of the sacral and lower lumbar nerve roots resulting from chronic adhesive arachnoiditis. It is associated with dural calcification and erosions of the spinal canal associated with enlarged dural sacs (dural ectasia) and dorsal dural diverticula that are characteristic of this condition and can be seen on CT and MRI. It causes sensory loss in the sacral and lower lumbar dermatomes ("saddle anesthesia") and decreased rectal or urinary sphincter tone, leading to disturbance of bowel and bladder function. It may also cause some pain and weakness in the legs. Myelopathy resembling multiple sclerosis has also been reported in AS patients, but epidemiological studies are needed to verify whether there is any association.[17]

Renal manifestations

Renal disease in AS can occur for various reasons. It presents with proteinuria and microscopic hematuria, sometimes detected on routine urinalysis, with or without impairment of renal function.[2,3] Secondary amyloidosis

(AA type) is now rarely observed among patients with AS or related SpA in the United States,[18] and the incidence is also decreasing in some other countries, possibly because of the more widespread use of NSAIDs and other drugs to control chronic inflammation. However, it often remains undiagnosed until late in its course because of its slow evolution and its relative rarity (≈1% of patients with chronic, poorly controlled inflammatory or infectious diseases). This complication should be considered in the differential diagnosis of proteinuria with or without progressive azotemia. An increased incidence of IgA nephropathy has also been reported, and renal impairment can sometimes result from NSAID use as well as from untreated hypertension.

Other possible associations

Some spondylitis patients with associated inflammatory bowel disease may develop pyoderma gangrenosum, erythema nodosum, or sclerosing cholangitis, the well-recognized extraintestinal manifestations of inflammatory bowel disease. Preliminary reports indicate that patients with AS and related SpA have an increased incidence of Sjögren's syndrome[19] and vitiligo.[20] A few cases of relapsing polychondritis[21] and retroperitoneal fibrosis[22] in patients with AS and related SpA have been reported.

References

1. Braun J, Sieper J. Ankylosing spondylitis. *Lancet.* 2007;369(9570):1379–1390.

2. Khan MA. Update on spondyloarthropathies. *Ann Intern Med.* 2002;136:896.

3. Khan MA. Ankylosing spondylitis: clinical features. In Hochberg M, Silman A, Smolen J, Weinblatt M, Weisman M, eds. *Rheumatology*, 3rd ed. London: Mosby: A Division of Harcourt Health Sciences Ltd.; 2003:1161–1181.

4. Zeboulon N, Dougados M, Gossec L. Prevalence and characteristics of uveitis in spondylarthropathies: a systematic literature review. *Ann Rheum Dis.* 2008;67(7):955–959.

5. Khan MA, Kushner I, Braun WE. Comparison of clinical features of HLA-B27 positive and negative patients with ankylosing spondylitis. *Arthritis Rheum.* 1977;20:909–912.

6. Lautermann D, Braun J. Ankylosing spondylitis—cardiac manifestations. *Clin Exp Rheumatol.* 2002;20(6 Suppl 28):S11–S15.

7. Quismorio FP Jr. Pulmonary involvement in ankylosing spondylitis. *Curr Opin Pulm Med.* 2006;12(5):342–345.

8. El Maghraoui A. Pleuropulmonary involvement in ankylosing spondylitis. *Joint Bone Spine.* 2005;72(6):496–502.

9. Bernstein CN, Blanchard JF, Rawsthorne P, Yu N. The prevalence of extraintestinal diseases in inflammatory bowel disease: a population based study. *Am J Gastroenterol.* 2001;96:1116–1122.

10. Smale S, Natt RS, Orchard TR, et al. Inflammatory bowel disease and spondylarthropathy. *Arthritis Rheum.* 2001;44:2728–2736.

11. De Vos M, Mielants H, Cuvelier C, et al. Long-term evolution of gut inflammation in patients with spondyloarthropathy. *Gastroenterology.* 1996;110:1696–1703.

12. Khan MA. Spondyloarthropathies. In Hunder G, ed. *Atlas of Rheumatology,* 4th ed. Philadelphia: Current Medicine; 2005:151–180.

13. Geusens P, Vosse D, van der Linden S. Osteoporosis and vertebral fractures in ankylosing spondylitis. *Curr Opin Rheumatol.* 2007;19(4):335–339.

14. Thumbikat P, Hariharan RP, Ravichandran G, McClelland MR, Mathew KM. Spinal cord injury in patients with ankylosing spondylitis: a 10-year review. *Spine.* 2007;32(26):2989–2995.

15. Fox MW, Onofrio BM, Kilgore JE. Neurological complications of ankylosing spondylitis. *J Neurosurg.* 1993;78(6):871–878.

16. Thompson GH, Khan MA, Bilenker RM. Spontaneous atlantoaxial subluxation as a presenting manifestation of juvenile ankylosing spondylitis. *Spine.* 1982;7:78–79.

17. Khan MA, Kushner I. Ankylosing spondylitis and multiple sclerosis: a possible association. *Arthritis Rheum.* 1979;22:784–786.

18. Ahmed Q, Chung-Park M, Mustafa K, Khan MA. Psoriatic spondyloarthropathy with secondary amyloidosis. *J Rheumatol.* 1996;23:1107–1110.

19. Kobak S, Kobak AC, Kabasakal Y, Doganavsargil E. Sjögren's syndrome in patients with ankylosing spondylitis. *Clin Rheumatol.* 2007;26(2):173–175.

20. Padula A, Ciancio G, La Civita L, et al. Association between vitiligo and spondyloarthritis. *J Rheumatol.* 2001;28(2):313–314.

21. Pazirandeh M, Ziran BH, Khandelwal BK, Reynolds TL, Khan MA. Relapsing polychondritis and spondyloarthropathies. *J Rheumatol.* 1988;15:630–632.

22. Afeltra A, Gentilucci UV, Rabitti C, et al. Retroperitoneal fibrosis and ankylosing spondylitis: which links? *Semin Arthritis Rheum.* 2005;35(1):43–48.

Chapter 9

Descriptions of related diseases: The spondyloarthropathies

The spondyloarthropathies (SpA) form a group of overlapping inflammatory rheumatologic diseases that show a tendency for involvement of the axial skeleton, entheses (bony insertions of ligaments and tendons; singular is "enthesis"), and peripheral joints (Fig. 1.4, Table 9.1). They may also show involvement of extraskeletal structures such as the eyes, skin, gut, and genitourinary tract.[1,2]

Table 9.1 Comparison of AS and related SpA

Characteristics	Disorders				
	AS	Reactive arthritis	Juvenile SpA	Psoriatic arthritis	Enteropathic SpA
Usual age at onset	Young adult age <40	Young to middle-aged	Ages 8 to 16 years	Young to middle age	Adult
Sex ratio	3x more common in males	Predominantly males	Predominantly males	Equal	Equal
Usual type of onset	Gradual	Acute	Variable	Variable	Gradual
Sacroiliitis or spondylitis	Virtually 100%	<50%	<50%	≈20%	<20%
Symmetry of sacroiliitis	Symmetric	Asymmetric	Variable	Asymmetric	Symmetric
Peripheral joint involvement	≈25%	≈90%	≈90%	≈95%	15% to 20%
HLA-B27 (in whites)	85% to 95%	40% to 80%	≈70%	<50%[‡]	≈50%[‡]
Eye involvement[§]	25% to 30%	≈50%	≈20%	≈20%	≤15%
Cardiac involvement	1% to 4%	5% to 10%	Rare	Rare	Rare
Skin or nail involvement	None	<40%	Uncommon	Virtually 100%	Uncommon
Role of infectious triggers	Unknown	Yes	Unknown	Unknown	Unknown

‡ HLA-B27 prevalence in those with spondylitis or sacroiliitis.

§ Predominantly conjunctivitis in reactive and psoriatic arthritis, and acute anterior uveitis in the other three disorders listed.

Reactive arthritis

Reactive arthritis (ReA) is an aseptic inflammatory arthritis that follows an episode of urethritis/cervicitis, diarrhea, or both. Inflammation may appear at sites other than the joints, such as the eyes, skin, and mouth.[1-3] The joint inflammation is caused by a bacterial infection that originates from a distant site, usually in the gastrointestinal or genitourinary tract, rather than the joint (Table 9.2). It classically occurs within 4 weeks after a triggering infection of the gut or the genitourinary tract, although many patients may not recall such a history. *Chlamydia trachomatis*, *Yersinia*, and *Salmonella* are the most relevant pathogens triggering ReA in developed countries. ReA, depending on the bacterial trigger, can be more common in men than in women.

Table 9.2 Infectious organisms associated with the onset of reactive arthritis

Enteric pathogens

Shigella flexneri, serotype 2a, 1b

Yersinia enterocolitica (serotypes 0:3, 0:8, 0:9)

   Y. pseudotuberculosis

Salmonella typhimurium

   S. enteritidis

   S. paratyphi

   S. heidelberg

   S. abony

   S. blocley

   S. schwarzengrund

   S. haifa

   S. manila

   S. newport

   S. bovismorbificans

Campylobacter jejuni

   C. fetus

Clostridium difficile

Vibrio parahemolyticus

Urogenital pathogens

Chlamydia trachomatis

   C. psittaci

?Ureaplasma urealyticum

Others

BCG intravesical injection for inoperable bladder cancer

C. pneumoniae

Not listed in the above table are reactive forms of arthritis following many bacterial (such as rheumatic fever), viral, and parasitic infections, as well as in association with intestinal bypass surgery, acne, hidradenitis suppurativa (abscesses in the armpit and groin), and cystic fibrosis, because they all lack any association with HLA-B27.

The prevalence of ReA in a population varies with the prevalence of HLA-B27 and that of the triggering bacterial infections. *Chlamydia*-induced ReA is most commonly seen in young, sexually active adults, mostly in males. However, it is underdiagnosed in women due to their frequently subclinical or asymptomatic chlamydial infection and the infrequency of pelvic examinations by physicians to look for the presence of cervicitis. The postenteritic form of the disease affects children and adults, both male and female, including the elderly.

The incidence of *Chlamydia*-induced ReA has declined since 1985 in Europe and the United States, while the incidence of the postenteritic form of the disease may be increasing. ReA occurs in about 1% to 4% of individuals following chlamydial urogenital infection. On the other hand, the incidence of ReA, or at least some form of musculoskeletal inflammation and pain, among HLA-B27-positive individuals in the general population after some epidemics of bacterial gastroenteritis or food poisoning (e.g., *Salmonella* enteritis) can be as high as 20%. The disease is more likely to become chronic or to be associated with acute iritis in HLA-B27-positive patients, but the initial episode of ReA in such epidemics is relatively weakly associated with HLA-B27 (no more than 33% of these patients may possess this gene).

Patients with ReA usually present with acute, asymmetrical oligoarthritis of the lower extremities; they also may have constitutional symptoms, urethritis, cervicitis, conjunctivitis, uveitis, genital lesions (circinate balanitis or vulvitis), keratoderma blennorrhagica, dactylitis, enthesitis, sacroiliitis/spondylitis, and nail discoloration and onycholysis without nail pitting.[1,2] The conjunctivitis is usually mild and bilateral and may not be noticed by the patient. It can cause eye irritation and redness, and sometimes the eyelids stick together in the morning. Some patients may have acute iritis. The classic triad of arthritis, conjunctivitis, and urethritis (formerly called Reiter's syndrome) may be present in a small subset of patients with this illness.

Acute episodes of ReA must be distinguished from other arthropathies that present in a similar fashion—septic arthritis, gout, pseudogout, juvenile arthritis, and sarcoid arthropathy, to name a few. Poststreptococcal ReA has been described in patients who do not meet the classification criteria for rheumatic fever.

Approximately 15% to 30% of patients develop chronic or recurrent arthritis, or sacroiliitis, or progress to spondylitis in later years. These patients are mostly those who are severely affected, have a positive family history for SpA, or are positive for HLA-B27. ReA in its chronic form can sometimes resemble PsA. The axial abnormalities are less common and less extensive than in AS, and involvement of the eyes (uveitis), cervical spine, and hip joints is less common. Sacroiliitis is often asymmetric or unilateral, and squaring of the vertebral bodies is less common than in AS. However, the axial disease in ReA is more often associated with peripheral arthritis than in primary AS. Tendinitis, enthesitis, or tenosynovitis can also occur alone or as focal or asymmetric oligoarticular involvement without resultant deformity. Inflammation, sometimes causing erosions or reactive bone formation, may occur in the sternoclavicular and manubriosternal joint and symphysis pubis.

Although the spondylitis of AS is generally a more widespread process, isolated involvement of the thoracic or lumbar spine may be the initial radiographic finding in the spine in reactive arthritis. Radiographic abnormalities of axial involvement are often asymmetric, with skip lesions that manifest as paravertebral ossifications and comma-shaped nonmarginal syndesmophytes (see Fig. 1.2f); they are often unilateral or asymmetric and tend to spare the anterior surface of the spine. Similar findings can occur in patients with psoriatic spondylitis.[1,2] They typically occur at the lower three thoracic and the lumbar vertebrae. Clinical enthesitis also tends to be asymmetric and is often more striking in the lower extremities (toes, calcaneus, tarsus, ankle, and knee).[1,2]

Severe disability occurs in fewer than 15% of patients and is often secondary to unrelenting lower extremity arthritis and enthesitis/dactylitis, aggressive axial involvement, or visual impairment. Death is rare, and in the past it was usually attributed to cardiac complications or amyloidosis. Bony ankylosis of peripheral joints is rarely observed.

Psoriatic arthritis

Psoriasis is a common chronic papulosquamous skin disease. It affects 2% to 3% of the U.S. population of European descent and is less common in blacks, Native Americans, and Southeast Asians. It is usually expressed in the form of itchy, dry, red, and scaly patches of skin; nails may show discoloration ("oil drop"), separation of distal nail plate from nail bed (onycholysis), pitting, and ridging. Several clinical phenotypes of psoriasis are recognized, with chronic plaque (psoriasis vulgaris) accounting for 90% of cases.

Comorbidities of psoriasis include PsA, conjunctivitis/iritis, impaired quality of life, stigmatization and associated depression, and adverse cardiovascular and metabolic outcomes. A new term, "psoriatic disease," encompasses these and other comorbidities observed in many psoriasis patients. PsA occurs in approximately 25% of psoriasis patients.[4] Its musculoskeletal characteristics include arthritis, dactylitis/sausage digits, enthesitis, tenosynovitis, and sacroiliitis/spondylitis.[2–8] Sausage-like diffuse swelling (dactylitis) of the toes or fingers ("sausage digits") and sometimes all of the joints in a single digit ("ray distribution") can occur.

Enthesitis at bony sites of attachment of ligaments and tendons can cause painful heels and tender back. Recalcitrant Achilles tendinitis/enthesitis and plantar fasciitis can also occur and may be predominant features.[5] In advanced stages of an uncommon subtype of PsA, severe resorption of the joints in the digits may occur; this can result in "telescoped" or collapsed digits and "opera glass" deformity in the fingers, but often not all joints are involved.[2–9]

Psoriatic spondylitis is clinically similar to AS, but it is more often associated with peripheral arthritis and less often with uveitis. There is often radiographic evidence of nonmarginal, large, asymmetrical syndesmophytes resembling those seen in ReA-associated spondylitis and sacroiliitis are often symptomatic, asymmetric, or unilateral (Fig. 1.2f).[2,6]

The polyarthritis form of PsA may resemble RA but has several characteristic features, including the involvement of the distal interphalangeal joints, dactylitis ("sausage digits"), periostitis, bony ankylosis, destructive "pencil-in-cup" deformities (a bone's distal head becomes pointed and the adjacent joint surface becomes cup-like because of erosions) in the fingers and toes, and nail involvement (discoloration, onycholysis, ridging, and especially pitting).[2,4,7,8] Conventional radiographs may reveal soft tissue swelling or erosive changes in the involved joints; a classic finding is periostitis, and juxtaarticular osteopenia, often seen in RA, is generally not a feature in PsA.

The onset of arthritis usually follows or coincides with the onset of psoriasis, although it antedates psoriasis in up to 15% of patients. The skin disease may not be readily apparent in some patients as it may be limited to the scalp, ears, umbilicus, perineum, and perianal area. Tissue-specific factors (biomechanical stressing and microdamage) related to the entheses, as well as genetic factors, play a role in triggering joint disease. Genetic studies suggest a multigenic mode of inheritance; a family history of psoriasis or PsA is present in up to 40% of patients with PsA. The disease affects men and women equally; onset usually occurs between 30 and 50 years of age, but the disease can begin in childhood. Evidence-based treatment guidelines have been published.[8]

Enteropathic SpA

Enteropathic SpA develops in up to 20% of patients with Crohn's disease or ulcerative colitis. It manifests as inflammatory back pain, enthesitis, or peripheral arthritis, fulfilling the ESSG criteria for SpA. Most of these patients with arthritis have peripheral joint inflammation that is usually nonerosive and correlates with flare-ups of bowel disease, especially in patients with ulcerative colitis. Up to 10% of patients fulfill the criteria for AS, with radiographic findings similar to those of primary AS; the axial disease does not correlate with bowel disease activity. Some patients have asymptomatic sacroiliitis.[3,10]

Subclinical inflammatory lesions in the gut have been observed in SpA patients without gut symptoms on ileocolonoscopy and mucosal biopsy. This gut inflammation in AS appears to be immunologically related to that seen in Crohn's disease in many of these patients. A similarly large percentage of patients with other forms of SpA have histologic gut inflammation.[10–13]

A long-term follow-up study of SpA patients with subclinical gut inflammation showed that full-blown inflammatory bowel disease developed in 7.3% of them. The presence of these Crohn's-like gut lesions is not associated with HLA-B27. These findings support the existence of a B27-independent common pathogenic link between gut inflammation and SpA.

Undifferentiated SpA

The term "undifferentiated SpA" is used when the patient has a limited form or early stage of the disease that does not meet the criteria for AS or the above-mentioned SpA that could be considered "differentiated" SpA.[3,14,15] Undifferentiated SpA encompasses disorders such as isolated enthesitis or dactylitis and RF-negative oligoarthritis or polyarthritis; it usually involves the lower extremities and often is HLA-B27-associated. Some patients may have episodes of acute anterior uveitis with one of the above-mentioned features but not psoriasis or gastrointestinal or genitourinary tract involvement, and they do not meet the ESSG criteria for SpA. In some patients with undifferentiated arthritis but with a joint pattern compatible with ReA, chlamydial DNA has been detected by polymerase chain reaction (PCR) in about 30% of cases in different countries. However, chlamydial DNA was rarely also found in control groups such as those with RA or healthy controls.

The undifferentiated form can occur in adults as well as children but is more commonly observed among children.[16] In fact, at least 50% of the time, SpA present in an undifferentiated form when they occur in childhood. Less than one-fourth of the children with AS or other "differentiated" types of SpA initially present with axial spine stiffness, restricted motion, or symptoms or signs of sacroiliitis. When a young child presents with isolated signs referable to the sacroiliac joint, infection, rather than SpA, might be a more appropriate diagnostic consideration. Sometimes leukemia and other forms of malignancy in children may mimic the clinical presentation of juvenile arthritis, including SpA.

Juvenile SpA

Juvenile or childhood-onset SpA refers to a group of SpA characterized by peripheral arthritis and enthesitis.[16] Sometimes the term "enthesitis-related arthritis" is used, referring to juvenile SpA in the juvenile idiopathic arthritis subgroup classification. These children may also have enthesitis and arthritis; this is sometimes called seronegative enthesitis and arthritis syndrome.

The disease may begin with enthesitis causing pain in the heels and other bony sites, or lower extremity arthritis of one (especially the knee or ankle) or a few joints. Most of these patients are boys ages 9 to 16 years, without any other features. This form of arthritis may precede the back pain by several years and may account for up to 20% of the whole group of juvenile chronic arthritis seen in pediatric rheumatology clinics. Intermittent episodes of pain in the groin and resultant limping, without any previous physical trauma or infection, can be a presenting manifestation, while other patients may present with enthesitis at multiple sites.

If the enthesitis affects the site of attachment of the patellar tendon into the tibial tubercle, a bony prominence an inch or so below the knee cap, it can be confused with Osgood-Schlatter's disease. However, children with juvenile SpA often also show tenderness at other bony sites due to enthesitis, not just at the tibial tubercles.

Patients with AS can also have a juvenile onset of their disease, and they complain of inflammatory back pain. However, radiographic sacroiliitis, one of the diagnostic hallmarks of SpA in adults, is not easy to detect in children. MRI is helpful in detecting sacroiliitis, especially in children and adolescents with clinical features suggestive of a spondyloarthropathy, because it can distinguish normal growth changes from true inflammatory disease, and it does not involve exposure to radiation.[17–19]

Many of these patients, especially among the Mexican Mestizo (of mixed genetic ancestry, mostly Native Americans with some Spanish admixture), present with undifferentiated SpA; severe enthesitis in the feet, in particular tarsitis, is the major feature that helps differentiate this SpA from other forms of juvenile idiopathic arthritis.[14] They also show a strong association with HLA-B27. Some of these children may develop juvenile-onset AS with back pain, sacroiliitis, and diminished spinal mobility. A study of such patients in Mexico has found that severe enthesitis in the feet is a common first presentation of AS in the Mestizo population.

ReA can also occur in children, usually triggered by enteric infection due to *Shigella*, *Salmonella*, or *Yersinia*. The arthritis is less severe than in adults, but as in adults, there is an association with HLA-B27. Juvenile onset of psoriatic arthritis is uncommon but well documented.

HIV-associated reactive arthritis

The HIV-associated form of ReA was first described in 1987 in the United States, when a group of patients were reported with both AIDS and severe arthritis or an illness resembling typical ReA, PsA, or undifferentiated SpA. In sub-Saharan Africa, due to the high prevalence of HIV infection, many patients are now being seen with these forms of SpA, which used to be rare among them.[1,20] For example, the prevalence of SpA in Lusaka, the capital of Zambia, a few years ago was calculated to be approximately 180 per 100,000 in HIV-infected individuals; this is 12 times higher than in the population unaffected with HIV.

The most common manifestations of HIV-associated ReA are arthralgia and arthritis; the latter is especially aggressive, and in many patients it develops after the patient becomes profoundly immunosuppressed. More than one-third of patients have an antecedent enteric or urogenital infection. Dactylitis, conjunctivitis, urethritis, psoriasis, recalcitrant enthesitis, and plantar fasciitis can also occur and sometimes predominate. The arthritis evolves in two main patterns: an additive, asymmetric polyarthritis, or an intermittent oligoarthritis that most commonly affects the lower extremities.[20] Although sacroiliitis is sometimes observed, axial spinal ankylosis is not observed, and acute anterior uveitis is rare. These patients are prone to bone and joint infections when their CD4+ T-cell count becomes markedly diminished. The arthritis differs from classical ReA not only in terms of the severity and chronicity of disease but also because of the relatively poor response to conventional drug therapy. However, efficacy of TNF antagonists has been reported in some HIV-positive patients with severe ReA.

The use of highly effective antiretroviral therapy in developed countries seems to have decreased the prevalence and expression of ReA and muco-cutaneous manifestations. HIV testing is not warranted in all patients suspected of having ReA in developed countries, but it may be considered in patients with ReA, PsA, or severe and relatively severe psoriasis who engage in high-risk behaviors or situations.

References

1. Khan MA, Sieper J. Reactive arthritis. In Koopman WJ, Moreland LW, eds. *Arthritis and Allied Conditions*, 15th ed. Philadelphia: Lippincott Williams & Wilkins; 2004:1335–1355.

2. Khan MA. Spondyloarthropathies. In Hunder G, ed. *Atlas of Rheumatology*, 4th ed. Philadelphia: Current Medicine; 2005:151–180.

3. Khan MA. Update on spondyloarthropathies. *Ann Intern Med*. 2002;36:896–907.

4. McCarey D, McInnes IB. Psoriatic arthritis: current topics. *Curr Rheumatol Rep*. 2007;9(6):442–448.

5. Gisondi P, Tinazzi I, El-Dalati G, et al. Lower limb enthesopathy in patients with psoriasis without clinical signs of arthropathy: a hospital-based case–control study. *Ann Rheum Dis*. 2008;67:26–30.

6. Gladman DD. Axial disease in psoriatic arthritis. *Curr Rheumatol Report*. 2007;9(6):455–460.

7. Taylor W, Gladman D, Helliwell P, et al. Classification criteria for psoriatic arthritis: development of new criteria from a large international study. *Arthritis Rheum*. 2006;54(8):2665–2673.

8. Kane D, Stafford L, Bresnihan B, FitzGerald O. A prospective, clinical and radiological study of early psoriatic arthritis: an early synovitis clinic experience. *Rheumatology (Oxford)*. 2003;42(12):1460–1468.

9. Kavanaugh A, Ritchlin CT, GRAPPA Treatment Guideline Committee. Systematic review of treatments for psoriatic arthritis: an evidence-based approach and basis for treatment guidelines. *J Rheumatol*. 2006;33(7):1417–1421.

10. Palm O, Moum B, Ongre A, Gran JT. Prevalence of ankylosing spondylitis and other spondyloarthropathies among patients with inflammatory bowel disease: a population study (the IBSEN study). *J Rheumatol*. 2002;29:511–515.

11. Bernstein CN, Blanchard JF, Rawsthorne P, Yu N. The prevalence of extraintestinal diseases in inflammatory bowel disease: a population-based study. *Am J Gastroenterol*. 2001;96:1116–1122.

12. Smale S, Natt RS, Orchard TR, et al. Inflammatory bowel disease and spondylarthropathy. *Arthritis Rheum*. 2001;44:2728–2736.

13. De Vos M, Mielants H, Cuvelier C, et al. Long-term evolution of gut inflammation in patients with spondyloarthropathy. *Gastroenterology*. 1996;110:1696–1703.

14. Burgos-Vargas R. Undifferentiated spondyloarthritis: a global perspective. *Curr Rheumatol Rep*. 2007;9(5):361–366.

15. Khan MA, van der Linden SM. A wider spectrum of spondyloarthropathies. *Semin Arthritis Rheum*. 1990;20:107–113.

16. Burgos-Vargas R. The juvenile-onset spondyloarthritides. *Rheum Dis Clin North Am.* 2002;28(3):531–560.

17. Weber U, Kissling JO, Hodler J. Advances in musculoskeletal imaging and their clinical utility in the early diagnosis of spondyloarthritis. *Curr Rheumatol Rep.* 2007;9(5):353–360.

18. Rudwaleit M, Khan MA, Sieper J. The challenge of diagnosis and classification in early ankylosing spondylitis: do we need new criteria? *Arthritis Rheum.* 2005;52:1000–1008.

19. van Tubergen A, Heuft-Dorenbosch L, Schulpen G, et al. Radiographic assessment of sacroiliitis by radiologists and rheumatologists: does training improve quality? *Ann Rheum Dis.* 2003;62(6):519–525.

20. Mijiyawa M, Oniankitan O, Khan MA. Spondyloarthropathies in sub-Saharan Africa. *Curr Opin Rheumatol.* 2000;12:263–268.

Chapter 10

Assessment of disease activity

It is important to distinguish symptoms that reflect active disease from symptoms of a mechanical or psychological nature before making specific treatment decisions.[1] Monitoring disease activity using reliable measures enables better assessment of response to treatment. C-reactive protein (CRP) and erythrocyte sedimentation rate (ESR) correlate only moderately with axial disease activity.[2-5] Several instruments have been developed to assess disease activity and severity of AS in a scoring system using symptoms and signs.[4-6]

BASDAI (Bath AS Disease Activity Index) is a reliable, easy-to-use, and sensitive-to-change measure that was designed by medical professionals in conjunction with patients.[7] It consists of seeking the patient's response to a self-administered questionnaire that contains six questions pertaining to the following five major symptoms of AS:

1. Fatigue and/or tiredness you have experienced
2. Axial musculoskeletal pain (spine, including neck and pelvis, and hip and shoulder girdles) you have had
3. Pain and/or swelling in other (peripheral) joints
4. Discomfort you have had from any areas tender to touch or pressure
5. Overall level of morning stiffness you have had from the time you wake up, and duration of morning stiffness

A visual analogue scale (VAS) that uses a horizontal line 10 cm in length or a numeric 0-to-10 scale (with 0 being the best and 10 being the worst) can be used to answer the questions. The patient is asked to give an average score during the preceding week. The BASDAI questionnaire form can be downloaded as PDF file from Ankylosing Spondylitis International Federation's (ASIF) Web site (www.spondylitis-international.org); it is found under "Practical forms for the assessment of AS." The questionnaire that uses a numeric scale is also available; it can be downloaded from www.asas-group.org, the Web site of Assessment of Spondyloarthritis International Society (ASAS).

There is one question each for the first four symptoms, and the fifth question relating to morning stiffness has two subcomponents (one for severity and the other for duration). Therefore, to give each symptom equal weighting, the average of the two scores relating to morning stiffness is calculated. The resulting total score of these five symptoms (the cal can range from 0 to 50) is divided by 5 to give a final BASDAI score, which can range from 0 to 10. Scores of 4 or more suggest suboptimal disease control; these patients may be good candidates for a change in their medical therapy, for treatment with biologic therapies, or for enrollment in clinical trials evaluating new drug therapies directed at AS. BASDAI needs to be used by rheumatologists and others who are familiar with fibromyalgia besides AS and related SpA; otherwise, patients with isolated or concomitant fibromyalgia will have a high BASDAI score that may not necessarily reflect the presence or inflammatory status of AS and related SpA.

BASFI (Bath AS Functional Index)[8] is also an easy, reliable, and sensitive-to-change method that assesses the degree of disability in patients with AS. It measures functional ability and coping skills on a 10 cm VAS and comprises 10 questions designed by medical professionals in conjunction with patients. The VAS anchors are labeled "easy" and "impossible." The BASFI questionnaire can be downloaded as PDF files from ASIF's Web site (www.spondylitis-international.org). The first eight questions consider activities related to functional abilities (e.g., putting on socks without help or aids), and the final two questions assess the patient's ability to cope with everyday life (e.g., doing a full day of activities at home or at work). BASFI scores can range from 0 to 10. Higher scores signify greater functional impairment. Another functional index, the Dougados Functional Index, is less popular.[9]

BASMI (Bath AS Metrology Index)[10] is a reproducible and sensitive method for assessing spinal mobility. It measures cervical extension using tragus-to-wall distance, lumbar flexion using the modified Schöber's test, cervical rotation using a goniometer, lumbar side flexion using fingertip-to-floor distance in sitting, and intermalleolar distance to measure bilateral hip abduction (Table 10.1). BASMI scores also range from 0 to 10; higher scores indicate greater impairment. A practical form for BASMI can be downloaded as PDF files from ASIF's Web site (www.spondylitis-international.org).

BASRI (Bath AS Radiology Index)[11] is a system of scoring radiographic change that combines the results of the BASRI–spine (which includes the scores of the sacroiliac joints and lumbar and cervical spine) and the BASRI–hip.

Table 10.1 Measuring mobility in AS: BASMI			
Score	0 = Mild impairment	1 = Moderate	2 = Severe
Tragus to wall	<15 cm	15 to 30 cm	>30 cm
Lumbar flexion	>4 cm	2 to 4 cm	<2 cm
Cervical rotation	>70 degrees	20 to 70 degrees	<20 degrees
Lumbar side flexion	>10 cm	5 to 10 cm	<5 cm
Intermalleolar distance	>100 cm	70 to 100 cm	<70 cm

mSASSS (modified Stoke AS Spondylitis Spine Score) is another radiologic scoring method[12] that offers advantages over BASRI for assessing the progression of structural damage in AS. It evaluates the anterior vertebral edges of the cervical and lumbar spine by grading the presence of chronic changes using a score of 0 (no damage) to 3 (bridging/syndesmophyte/ankylosis), with total scores ranging between 0 and 72. Definite radiographic progression is defined as a change in mSASSS from 0 or 1 (suspicious damage) to >2 (syndesmophytes or ankylosis). However, there is still a need for a better scoring method because mSASSS focuses heavily on the formation of syndesmophytes and the occurrence of ankylosis (osteoproliferation), while erosive changes (osteolysis) have a minor influence on the total score. A practical form for mSASSS and BASRI can be downloaded as PDF files from ASIF's Web site (www.spondylitis-international.org).

Other validated measures of disease outcome[4–6,13,14] include the following:

- **SF-36** (Medical Outcomes Short-Form 36) is a self-administered questionnaire that assesses eight domains of quality of life: physical functioning, pain, role limitations due to physical problems, role limitations due to emotional problems, mental health, social functioning, energy/fatigue, and general health perceptions.

- **HAQ** (Health Assessments Questionnaire) is a tool to evaluate functional disability and can be modified to assess spondylitis-specific measures (HAQ-S).[15] It has also been modified to assess the severity of psoriatic arthritis.[16]

- **MFI** (Multidimensional Fatigue Inventory) is a 20-item self-report instrument to measure fatigue. It covers general, physical, and mental fatigue and reduced motivation/activity.

- **FACIT** (Functional Assessment of Chronic Illness Therapy), fourth version, is a 13-item composite scale that is used to evaluate fatigue. It uses a cross-cultural approach.

Assessment of clinical disease severity

Clinical assessment of disease severity in patients with AS is sometimes difficult, especially in uncomplicated early disease that is confined to the sacroiliac joints and spine.[4–6] Useful parameters to assess disease severity in AS include structural damage assessed by radiographs, metrological evaluation such as BASFI, BASMI, and presence of hip joint involvement and extraarticular manifestations. As discussed earlier, the useful parameters to assess disease activity in AS include BASDAI, overall pain, pain at night, patient's global assessment, ESR and CRP, daily function (BASFI, working ability), extraarticular manifestations, and peripheral arthritis. MRI of the sacroiliac joints or spine can be considered in selected cases to assess the extent of inflammatory lesions.

Assessment of response of disease activity to treatment

ASAS response criteria

The ASAS working group has developed ASAS response criteria with 20% improvement (ASAS20), 50% improvement (ASAS50), or 70% improvement (ASAS70) as measure of short-term improvement in AS; these criteria have both clinical and empirical validity.[4–6,14] The ASAS20, -50, and -70 response criteria are designed to be used as summary outcome measures in clinical trials.

The ASAS20 response, which was developed on the basis of clinical trials with NSAIDs,[4,14] is defined as an improvement of at least 20% and absolute improvement of at least 10 units (on a scale of 0 to 100) in three of the following four domains: patient global assessment, pain, inflammation (mean of the last two BASDAI questions), and function (BASFI) (Table 10.2). There must also be absence of deterioration in the potential remaining domain (deterioration defined as at least 20% worsening and net worsening of at least 10 units on a scale of 0 to 100).

The ASAS50 and ASAS70 response criteria have the same definition, except that they require an improvement of at least 50% and at least 70%, respectively, in three of the four domains. They are more suitable than ASAS20 for demonstrating efficacy of TNF antagonists.

An ASAS5/6 response is similar to the ASAS20 response, except that it contains two more components: the BASMI score and CRP. It requires achieving at least a 20% improvement in five of its six domains and absence of deterioration in the potentially remaining sixth domain.[4–7] This level of response is more useful for assessing improvement in clinical trials of drugs such as TNF antagonists in AS, and is now considered the preferred primary target in clinical efficacy trials in AS.

Patient Acceptable Symptom State (PASS)

A recently described concept, Patient Acceptable Symptom State (PASS), is reliable and valid for assessing the health of AS patients.[17,18] It is assessed by asking patients to respond yes or no to a single question: "Considering

---

Table 10.2 ASAS20 response criteria

An improvement of ≥20% and absolute improvement of ≥10 units on a 0-to-100 scale in at least three of the following four domains:

1. Patient global assessment (by VAS global assessment)
2. Pain assessment (average of VAS total and nocturnal pain scores)
3. Function (represented by BASFI)
4. Inflammation (the average of the BASDAI's last two VAS concerning morning stiffness: intensity and duration)

and

Absence of deterioration in the potential remaining domain (deterioration is defined as 20% worsening) all the different ways your disease is affecting you, if you would stay in this state for the next months, do you consider that your current state is satisfactory?" The PASS scores, defined as the 75th percentile of the score for patients who considered their state satisfactory and shown on a 0-to-10 scale (10 being worst), are reported to be 3.4 for global pain, 2.8 for night pain, 3.6 for patient's global disease assessment, 3.5 for BASDAI, and 3.1 for BASFI.[17]

Disease remission

Just as disease remission is now the accepted goal of management of RA, it is being increasingly regarded as an appropriate therapeutic goal for AS because of the availability of more effective therapies.[1,5,13] Early use of TNF-antagonist therapy in RA has been shown to lead to significant improvement in disease activity measures; that improvement is sustained in a high percentage of patients 1 year after stopping treatment. This suggests that early use of TNF-blocking therapy can produce a sustainable remission in some patients with early RA without the need for long-term administration. This has important implications for health economics, and studies need to be performed to see if a similar result can be achieved in patients with early AS. This will also require defining the criteria for remission, which will include clinical, immunological, and imaging assessments. Furthermore, based on studies of anti-TNF therapy in AS, a state of low disease activity has been suggested empirically, but it needs further development and evaluations for defining a state of "true" disease remission in AS.[13] An ASAS criterion for partial remission has been proposed that requires that each of the four domains of ASAS20 be under 2 on a 0-to-10 scale.[14]

Composite core set for use in daily practice

A composite core set for clinical and functional assessment of AS has been developed for use in daily practice.[5,19] Table 10.3 shows the ASAS core

Table 10.3 ASAS core set for evaluation of disease-controlling antirheumatic treatment (DCART)	
Domains	**Instruments**
Physical function	BASFI (or Dougados Functional Index)
Pain	Total pain in the spine due to AS in the past week, VAS (0-to-100 scale)
	Night pain in the spine due to AS in the past week, VAS (0-to-100 scale)
Spinal mobility	Chest expansion
	Modified Schober's test
	Occiput-to-wall distance
	Lateral spinal flexion or BASMI

Table 10.3 *continued*	
Domains	**Instruments**
Spinal stiffness	Duration of morning stiffness in the spine in the past week
Patient global assessment	VAS (0-to-100 scale), past week
Peripheral joints/entheses	Number of swollen joints (44 joint count); currently no preferred instruments available for entheses
Acute phase reactants	Erythrocyte sedimentation rate
Spine radiograph	AP + lateral lumbar and lateral cervical spine
Hip radiograph	Radiograph of the pelvis (sacroiliac joint and hips)
Fatigue	VAS (0-to-100 scale), past week

set for evaluation of disease-controlling antirheumatic therapies (DCART). The first five of these components (physical function, pain, spinal mobility, patient global, and spinal stiffness) make up the core set for symptom-modifying antirheumatic therapy and physical therapy (SMART/PT) in AS. The components for clinical recordkeeping are the first five components plus peripheral joints, entheses, and acute phase reactants.

References

1. Khan MA. Ankylosing spondylitis: burden of illness, diagnosis, and effective treatment. *J Rheumatol Suppl.* 2006;78:1–33.

2. Ozgocmen S, Godekmerdan A, Ozkurt-Zengin. Acute-phase response, clinical measures and disease activity in ankylosing spondylitis. *Joint Bone Spine.* 2007;74(3):249–253.

3. Spoorenberg A, van der Heijde D, de Klerk E, et al. Relative value of erythrocyte sedimentation rate and C-reactive protein in assessment of disease activity in ankylosing spondylitis. *J Rheumatol.* 1999;26(4):980–984.

4. Zochling J, Braun J. Assessment of ankylosing spondylitis. *Clin Exp Rheumatol.* 2005;23(5 suppl 39):S133–S141.

5. Zochling J, Braun J, van der Heijde D. Assessments in ankylosing spondylitis. *Best Pract Res Clin Rheumatol.* 2006;20(3):521–537.

6. Sengupta R, Stone MA. The assessment of ankylosing spondylitis in clinical practice. *Nat Clin Pract Rheumatol.* 2007;3(9):496–503.

7. Garrett S, Jenkinson T, Kennedy LG, Whitelock H, Gaisford P, Calin A. A new approach to defining disease status in ankylosing spondylitis: the Bath Ankylosing Spondylitis Disease Activity Index. *J Rheumatol.* 1994;21(12):2286–2291.

8. Calin A, Garrett S, Whitelock H, et al. A new approach to defining functional ability in ankylosing spondylitis: the development of the Bath Ankylosing Spondylitis Functional Index. *J Rheumatol.* 1994;21(12):2281–2285.

9. Dougados M, Gueguen A, Nakache JP, Nguyen M, Mery C, Amor B. Evaluation of a functional index and an articular index in ankylosing spondylitis. *J Rheumatol.* 1988;15(2):302–307.

10. Jenkinson TR, Mallorie PA, Whitelock HC, Kennedy LG, Garrett SL, Calin A. Defining spinal mobility in ankylosing spondylitis (AS). The Bath AS Metrology Index. *J Rheumatol.* 1994;21(9):1694–1698.

11. MacKay K, Mack C, Brophy S, Calin A. The Bath Ankylosing Spondylitis Radiology Index (BASRI): a new, validated approach to disease assessment. *Arthritis Rheum.* 1998;41(12):2263–2270.

12. Salaffi F, Carotti M, Garofalo G, Giuseppetti GM, Grassi W. Radiological scoring methods for ankylosing spondylitis: a comparison between the Bath Ankylosing Spondylitis Radiology Index and the modified Stoke Ankylosing Spondylitis Spine Score. *Clin Exp Rheumatol.* 2007;25(1):67–74.

13. Zochling J, Braun J. Remission in ankylosing spondylitis. *Clin Exp Rheumatol.* 2006;24(6 Suppl 43):S88–S92.

14. Anderson JJ, Baron G, van der Heijde D, Felson DT, Dougados M. Ankylosing spondylitis assessment group preliminary definition of short-term improvement in ankylosing spondylitis. *Arthritis Rheum.* 2001;44(8):1876–1886.

15. Doward LC, Spoorenberg A, Cook SA, et al. Development of the ASQoL: a quality of life instrument specific to ankylosing spondylitis. *Ann Rheum Dis.* 2003;62(1):20–26.

16. McKenna SP, Doward LC, Whalley D, Tennant A, Emery P, Veale DJ. Development of the PsAQoL: a quality of life instrument specific to psoriatic arthritis. *Ann Rheum Dis.* 2004;63(2):162–169.

17. Tubach F, Pham T, Skomsvall JF, et al. Stability of the patient acceptable symptomatic state over time in outcome criteria in ankylosing spondylitis. *Arthritis Rheum.* 2006; 55(6):960–963.

18. Dougados M, Luo MP, Maksymowych WP, et al. Evaluation of the patient acceptable symptom state as an outcome measure in patients with ankylosing spondylitis: data from a randomized controlled trial. *Arthritis Rheum.* 2008;59(4):553–560.

19. van der Heijde D, Calin A, Dougados M, Khan MA, van der Linden S, Bellamy N. Selection of instruments in the core set for DC-ART, SMARD, physical therapy, and clinical record keeping in ankylosing spondylitis. Progress report of the ASAS Working Group. Assessments in Ankylosing Spondylitis. *J Rheumatol.* 1999;26(4):951–954.

Chapter 11

Disease management

The treatment of AS should be individualized based on the disease activity and severity and the patient's symptoms and signs, functional status, deformities, general health status, comorbid conditions, and wishes.[1] The best strategy incorporates patient and family education; lifestyle and workplace modifications; physical therapy; a lifelong program of regular physical exercise; use of medications; when appropriate, referral to appropriate specialists; and monitoring of disease activity and adverse effects of drug therapies.[1–4]

Evidence-based guidelines for management of patients with AS

Evidence-based guidelines have been developed by the Assessment in AS International Working Group (ASAS) and the European League Against Rheumatism (EULAR) to assist health-care professionals involved in the care of patients with AS.[3] These guidelines are listed below, and the flow chart is shown in Figure 11.1.

1. Treatment of AS should be tailored according to the current disease manifestations, the level of current symptoms, clinical findings and prognostic indicators, and the patient's wishes and expectations.

2. Disease monitoring should include patient history, which may be documented using questionnaires; clinical parameters, laboratory tests, and imaging (as indicated based on the clinical presentation); and the ASAS core set.

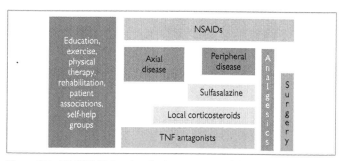

Figure 11.1 ASAS/EULAR flowchart for the management of ankylosing spondylitis. Reprinted, with permission from Wolters Kluwer Health, from Boulos P, Dougados M, Macleod SM, Hunsche E. Pharmacological treatment of ankylosing spondylitis: a systematic review. *Drugs.* 2005;65:2111–2127.

3. Optimal management of AS mandates a combination of nonpharmacological and pharmacological treatment.

4. Nonpharmacological AS management should include patient education and regular exercise, with consideration of individual and group physical therapy, patient associations, and self-help groups.

5. NSAIDs are first-line drug treatment for patients with AS with pain and stiffness. For patients with a higher risk for gastrointestinal tract complications, nonselective NSAIDs plus a gastroprotective agent or a selective cycclooxygenase-2 inhibitor could be used.

6. Paracetamol, opioids, or other analgesics may be considered for pain control in patients in whom NSAIDs are insufficient, contraindicated, or poorly tolerated.

7. Corticosteroid injections directed to the local site of musculoskeletal inflammation may be considered, but the use of systemic corticosteroids for axial disease is not supported by the available evidence.

8. There is no evidence for the efficacy of disease-modifying antirheumatic drugs (DMARDs), including sulfasalazine (SSZ) and methotrexate (MTX), for the treatment of axial disease. However, SSZ may be considered for patients with peripheral arthritis.

9. Patients with persistently high disease activity despite conventional treatments should receive treatment with TNF antagonists. In patients with axial disease, there is no evidence to support the mandatory use of DMARDs before or concomitant with anti-TNF treatment.

10. Total hip arthroplasty should be considered in patients with refractory pain or disability and radiographic evidence of structural damage, regardless of age. In selected patients, spinal surgery (corrective osteotomy or stabilization procedures) may be indicated.

The 3E (Evidence, Experts, Exchange) Initiative in Rheumatology, a multinational effort of rheumatologists with a special interest in clinical research, comprises 12 key evidence-based statements (recommendations) for the diagnosis, monitoring, and treatment of AS to facilitate translating research into practice without restricting the autonomy of treating physicians.[4] These 12 statements are listed below. Three of them address general diagnostic considerations, early AS diagnosis, and general practitioners' referral recommendations; another three concern monitoring of AS disease activity, severity, and prognosis; and the remaining six concern pharmacological treatment (except biologics): NSAIDs/COX-2 inhibitors, bisphosphonates, and treatment of enthesitis. The compiled agreement among experts ranged from 72% to 93%. Longitudinal studies will be needed to document the effect of these recommendations in reducing health-care-related costs and curbing unjustified variations in clinical practice.

1. In chronic back pain of at least 3 months' duration, the presence of several of the following features makes the diagnosis of AS likely: inflammatory back pain, alternating buttock pain, response to NSAIDs, onset of symptoms before age 45, peripheral disease manifestations (arthritis,

dactylitis, enthesitis), confirmed acute anterior uveitis, positive family history, HLA-B27 positive, sacroiliitis/spondylitis by imaging.

2. For early diagnosis of AS, no additional imaging is required if definite radiographic changes of sacroiliitis are present. If radiographs of the sacroiliac joints are normal or equivocal, MRI is the best imaging modality to identify inflammation of the sacroiliac joints and spine. CT is a sensitive tool for identifying structural changes of the sacroiliac joints, but the risks of radiation exposure need to be considered.

3. Patients with chronic back pain of at least 3 months' duration and features of inflammatory back pain (onset of symptoms before age 45 years, back pain at night, morning stiffness and improvement with exercise) should be referred to a rheumatologist for further evaluation of possible AS.

4. Useful parameters to assess disease *activity* in AS include BASDAI, overall pain, pain at night, patient's global assessment, erythrocyte sedimentation rate (ESR) and/or C-reactive protein (CRP), daily function (BASFI, working ability), extraarticular manifestations, and peripheral arthritis. MRI of the sacroiliac joints and/or spine can be considered in selected cases.

5. Useful parameters to assess disease *severity* in AS include structural damage assessed by radiographs, metrological evaluation such as BASMI, measures of function such as BASFI, hip involvement, and extraarticular manifestations.

6. Predictors of a poor prognosis in AS Include radiographic structural changes of the spine at initial assessment, hip involvement, young age at disease onset, persistently elevated acute phase reactants, and persistently high disease activity.

7. There are insufficient data to support the use of bisphosphonates in the treatment of active AS. However, bisphosphonates may be useful for the management of osteoporosis in AS.

8. NSAIDs can be used for the treatment of enthesitis in patients with AS. Local corticosteroid injections may be the preferred treatment in selected cases.

9. NSAIDs are the first-line treatment for relief of pain and improvement of daily function in AS. NSAIDs should be used as needed in AS for symptoms of active disease. There is no significant difference in efficacy between short-acting and long-acting agents or between COX-2 selective and nonselective agents.

10. AS patients with persistently active disease may require continuous use of NSAIDs, but this may increase the risk of side effects, including cardiovascular toxicity. In patients at higher risk for gastrointestinal side effects, a selective COX-2 agent, or a nonselective NSAID in combination with a gastroprotective agent, should be considered.

11. NSAIDs are effective for axial, peripheral, and entheseal features of AS, although axial symptoms are most responsive.

12. There is limited evidence that NSAID use in AS precipitates first presentations of IBD or flares of preexisting disease. IBD patients treated with NSAIDs should be monitored closely by both the prescribing doctor and a gastroenterologist.

Nonpharmacological treatment

Nonpharmacological modalities complement drug therapy and are important in all stages of the disease in both axial and peripheral involvement.

Patient education

Patients should be provided with disease-specific written instructions and illustrations, handouts, books, pamphlets, videos, audiotapes, and information about useful Web sites (see Appendix 1).[2,5] All patients should receive instructions on proper posture and appropriate home-based exercises, and they should be encouraged to perform water exercises if they can. Self-help programs and patient education and counseling improve patients' compliance with therapy regimens and benefit their general health and functional status. Cessation of cigarette smoking should be strongly encouraged because smoking is associated with worse outcomes. Patients also should receive pneumococcal and yearly influenza vaccinations, especially when treatment with TNF-α inhibitors is being considered.

Patients' posture problems and difficulties in performing activities of daily living should be identified, and workplace modifications may be needed. Frequently changing position when sitting at a desk and taking breaks for body stretching are helpful. Activities that cause back muscle strain should be avoided (e.g., prolonged stooping or bending and assuming positions that may cause a stooped posture, such as prolonged slouching in chairs or leaning over a desk). Helpful assistive devices include long-handled devices for dressing and for reaching or picking objects, adjustable swivel chairs that provide lumbar support, and elevated and inclined writing surfaces. Use of wide-view mirrors can be helpful for patients with limited neck mobility when driving. Use of back splints, braces, and corsets is not helpful and should be avoided.

Exercise and physical therapy

Data on the role of exercise and physical therapy are limited in terms of the duration of follow-up, and specific treatment protocols have not been thoroughly studied. Regular exercise and formal sessions of physical therapy are generally underused by patients and physicians. These nonpharmacological modalities remain an essential part of the management plan, despite the remarkable progress in the pharmacological therapy of AS. They complement drug therapy to improve function and quality of life and to minimize deformities.[2–4,6,7] They may have other benefits as well, including less pain, better mood, and improved quality of life and health status, as well as maintenance or improvement in posture, chest expansion, and lung vital capacity. They are of fundamental importance for the successful long-term management of patients with AS, so physicians should educate patients about the role of exercise and give them instructions about simple exercises. Patients should be referred to a physical therapist for specific exercise instructions for spinal extension, deep breathing, and range-of-motion exercises of the back, neck, shoulders, hips, and other joints.

Home-based exercise programs are easily performed and are convenient and free. Patients who participate in a regular long-term exercise program may show improvement in exercise self-effectiveness, mobility, and function. Formal physical therapy and, in the most severe cases, inpatient rehabilitation may be needed in select patients with severe AS. Patients who undergo supervised group physical therapy combined with comprehensive home exercises supported by educational interventions have shown improved spinal mobility and function that can be sustained with maintenance exercises. A yearly follow-up visit to a physiotherapist can ensure that these exercises are being performed appropriately; this can also keep track of any improvement or worsening in physical posture and joint and spine range of motion.

High-impact and contact sports activities and those that involve abrupt movement of the spine should be avoided, especially by patients who have axial disease with limited spinal mobility. Back stretching and deep breathing exercises, swimming and water aerobics, stationary bicycling, and other appropriate recreational exercises are especially useful. They can help enhance general fitness, lung capacity, exercise capability, muscle strength, and range of motion. They also increase cardiovascular conditioning and endurance. Patients with heart disease should be assessed by their physician and may require an exercise tolerance test before starting to exercise.

Patients usually feel that their back is too stiff to exercise in the morning, so they can choose a time of the day that works best for them. A warm shower before exercising tends to ease discomfort during exercise, promotes relaxation, and helps in passive stretching of tight muscles. Therapeutic exercises must be tailored to the patient's degree of spinal mobility or involvement, and they should ideally be performed routinely.

A heated swimming pool or a spa helps to decrease pain and stiffness and therefore allows the patient to perform exercises that might be otherwise impossible because of pain and stiffness. Regular freestyle swimming is considered to be one of the best exercises for AS patients. The patient must be careful not to slip on the wet surfaces in the pool area, and also it is wise to avoid diving. It may be difficult for patients with rigid necks to swim freestyle, although the use of a snorkel may be helpful, provided the patient swims only under observation and near the edge of a swimming pool if it is deep. This precaution is necessary because patients with limited breathing capacity may not be able to blow out the water if it inadvertently enters the snorkel tube. In some European countries, professionally supervised special physiotherapy and hydrotherapy group sessions for AS patients have been organized by AS patient societies, and group exercise sessions at a spa or hydrotherapy center are enjoyable and very helpful. Patients with psoriasis should avoid chlorinated water.

Pharmacological treatment

NSAIDs

NSAIDs are still the first-line drug therapy for patients with active AS. Both traditional as well as selective COX-2 inhibitors have been shown to decrease axial and peripheral joint pain and improve function.[1–4,8–11] NSAIDs need to be taken regularly in full anti-inflammatory doses to achieve the desired therapeutic effect.

More than 20 types of NSAIDs are available. Some of the NSAIDs available in the United States are listed in Table 11.1. Brand names may vary in different parts of the world.

The various NSAIDs are of comparable efficacy, but there are individual variations in response of AS patients to different NSAIDs, in addition to variations in their side effect profiles and drug interactions.[4,8–11] Therefore, some patients may need to try other NSAIDs to find the most effective one before giving up on them for disease management. NSAIDs may also

Table 11.1 Non-aspirin NSAIDs marketed in the United States

Brand name	Generic name
Anaprox DS	Naproxen sodium
Ansaid	Flurbiprofen
Arthrotec	Diclofenac plus misoprostol
Celebrex	Celecoxib
Clinoril	Sulindac
Daypro	Oxaprozin
Dolobid	Diflunisal
Feldene	Piroxicam
Indocin (Indocid)	Indomethacin
Lodine	Etodolac
Mobic	Meloxicam
Motrin	Ibuprofen
Naprosyn	Naproxen
Orudis	Ketoprofen
Relafen	Nabumetone
Tolectin	Tolmetin sodium
Toradol	Ketorolac tromethamnine
Voltaren	Diclofenac sodium
Ponstel	Mefenamic acid
Meclomen	Meclofenamate
Nalfon	Fenoprofen
Salsalate	Disalcid
Trilisate	Choline magnesium trisalicylate
Todolac	Etodolac

be effective in ReA as well as mild peripheral PsA, when there is no evidence of erosions.

In few case reports, treatment with nonselective NSAIDs in IBD patients has been reported to lead to frequent disease exacerbation, but selective COX-2 inhibitors may be better tolerated. However, there is limited evidence that NSAID use in AS precipitates first presentations of IBD or flares of preexisting disease.[4] However, IBD patients treated with NSAIDs should be monitored closely by both the prescribing doctor and a gastroenterologist.

The risk of gastrointestinal bleeding is dose-dependent; selective COX-2 inhibitors carry a lower risk of serious gastrointestinal events than nonselective (traditional) NSAIDs. Another way to reduce the risk for gastrointestinal complications is to avoid smoking and alcohol intake and to use a gastrointestinal-protective agent such as misoprostol or a proton pump inhibitor. The cardiovascular toxicity seen with rofecoxib (Vioxx), which was taken off the market, has also been described in clinical trials of other selective COX-2 inhibitors, with some evidence suggesting that it may be an NSAIDs class effect. However, a recent meta-analysis did not reveal an increased risk of cardiovascular events with celecoxib.[4,12]

NSAIDs do to some extent inhibit osteoproliferation, possibly by inhibiting prostaglandins (see Chapter 12). There is preliminary evidence that regular therapy with an NSAID compared to as-needed use may have a mild disease-modifying effect, as shown by retarding the radiographic progression of the disease.[4,13,14] NSAIDs decrease heterotopic bone formation after hip replacement surgery, but this favorable effect should be weighed against possible adverse effects such as bleeding or impaired bone healing.

Other drugs

The traditional DMARDs, such as MTX, leflunomide, and SSZ, are not recommended for managing axial disease because they have not been proven to be efficacious in its treatment of axial disease.[3,4,15–18] SSZ may be tried in patients with predominantly peripheral arthritis at a dose that is gradually increased over many days from 1 g daily to a maximum tolerated dose of 2 g or preferably 3 g per day. Adverse effects of SSZ are common and include gastrointestinal upset, skin rashes, and hepatic and hematological toxicities.

Oral corticosteroids are not recommended in axial disease because of lack of benefit and significant side effects. However, local or intraarticular corticosteroid injections can be used in some patients to achieve rapid relief of enthesitis and monoarticular or oligoarticular peripheral arthritis in the absence of contraindications. Sacroiliitis pain has been shown to improve with intra- or periarticular steroid injections in some patients, but the beneficial effect is not very prolonged.[19–21] Topical corticosteroids are very effective for the treatment of acute iritis. Options to prevent recurrences of acute iritis associated with AS include the use of SSZ, but TNF antagonists, especially monoclonal antibodies, are much more effective in preventing recurrence of uveitis.

A 12-month open-label trial of thalidomide showed efficacy in 80% of 26 Chinese males with AS.[22] The benefit was noted gradually over the first few months, with at least 20% improvement in four of seven outcome measures, and was sustained for many weeks after the end of the study. Its well-known teratogenic effects require absolute prevention of pregnancy; severe sedation and the risk of irreversible neuropathy are other limiting factors.

There are insufficient data to support the use of bisphosphonates in the treatment of active AS.[3] Pamidronate, a bisphosphonate given at a dose of 60 mg by intravenous infusion once a month, was shown to reduce disease activity, both clinically and on MRI scanning, but the benefit was very modest at best and there was no reduction in ESR or CRP.[23] However, bisphosphonates may be useful for the management of osteoporosis in AS, which is quite common and should be recognized and managed early.

Osteopenia and osteoporosis can occur relatively early in the disease process, as it is caused in part by the ankylosis and resultant decreased mobility; it can also be secondary to the effect of the proinflammatory cytokines. Prevention and treatment of osteoporosis may help decrease the risk of deformities and fractures and the morbidity and mortality associated with them.

Measurements of bone density at the spine may be unreliable when there is ligamentous ossification and formation of syndesmophytes. Thus, femoral neck measurements should be relied on for the diagnosis. A peripheral DEXA scan might have to be relied on in patients with bilateral hip arthroplasties. Vitamin D deficiency should be screened for and corrected if present. Adequate intake of calcium and vitamin D should be ensured; the recommended daily intake is 1.0 to 1.5 g of elemental calcium and 400 to 800 IU of vitamin D.

In some patients, simple analgesics such as acetaminophen and tramadol may be used as adjunctive short-term treatment until the inflammation is controlled by other means. Caution should be exercised when prescribing narcotics in such situations because of the risk of dependence and abuse. Low-dose tricyclic agents such as amitriptyline (Elavil) may be a helpful adjunctive treatment to relieve pain and fatigue, especially in patients with sleep disturbances, but it may cause some untoward effects, such as drowsiness and dryness of the mouth.

There is no role for a special diet or use of antibiotics for the treatment of AS. Patients with *Chlamydia*-induced ReA and their sexual partners may need to be treated simultaneously with appropriate antibiotics to eradicate the infection, although such treatment may not alter the natural disease course of ReA.[24]

References

1. Khan MA. Ankylosing spondylitis: burden of illness, diagnosis, and effective treatment. *J Rheumatol Suppl.* 2006;78:1–33.

2. Khan MA. *Ankylosing Spondylitis: The Facts.* Oxford: Oxford University Press; 2002.

3. Zochling J, van der Heijde D, Burgos-Vargas R, et al. ASAS/EULAR recommendations for the management of ankylosing spondylitis. *Ann Rheum Dis.* 2006;65:442–452.

4. Sidiropoulos PI, Hatemi G, Song IH, et al. Evidence-based recommendations for the management of ankylosing spondylitis: systematic literature search of the 3E Initiative in Rheumatology involving a broad panel of experts and practising rheumatologists. *Rheumatology (Oxford)*. 2008;47(3):355–361.

5. Feldtkeller E, Bruckel J, Khan MA. Scientific contributions of the ankylosing spondylitis patient advocacy groups. *Curr Opin Rheumatol*. 2000;12:239–247.

6. Elyan M, Khan MA. The role of non-steroidal anti-inflammatory medications and exercise in the treatment of ankylosing spondylitis. *Curr Rheumatol Report*. 2006;8:255–259.

7. Elyan M, Khan MA. Does physical therapy have a place in the treatment of ankylosing spondylitis? *Curr Opin Rheumatol*. 2008;20(3):282–286.

8. Song IH, Poddubnyy DA, Rudwaleit M, Sieper J. Benefits and risks of ankylosing spondylitis treatment with nonsteroidal antiinflammatory drugs. *Arthritis Rheum*. 2008;58(4):929–938.

9. Khan MA. A double-blind comparison of dicloflenac and indomethacin in the treatment of ankylosing spondylitis. *J Rheumatol*. 1987;14:118–123.

10. Sieper J, Klopsch T, Richter M, et al. Comparison of two different dosages of celecoxib with diclofenac for the treatment of active ankylosing spondylitis: results of a 12-week randomised, double-blind, controlled study. *Ann Rheum Dis*. 2008;67(3):323–329.

11. Boulos P, Dougados M, Macleod SM, Hunsche E. Pharmacological treatment of ankylosing spondylitis: a systematic review. *Drugs*. 2005;65:2111–2127.

12. White WB, West CR, Borer JS, et al. Risk of cardiovascular events in patients receiving celecoxib: a meta-analysis of randomized clinical trials. *Am J Cardiol*. 2007;99:91–98.

13. Wanders A, Heijde D, Landewé R, et al. Inhibition of radiographic progression in ankylosing spondylitis (AS) by continuous use of NSAIDs. *Arthritis Rheum*. 2005;52(6):1756–1765.

14. Ward MM. Prospects for disease modification in ankylosing spondylitis: do non-steroidal antiinflammatory drugs do more than treat symptoms? *Arthritis Rheum*. 2005;52(6):1634–1636.

15. Haibel H, Brandt HC, Song HI, et al. No efficacy of subcutaneous methotrexate in active ankylosing spondylitis: a 16-week open-label trial. *Ann Rheum Dis*. 2007;66(3):419–421.

16. Chen J, Liu C, Lin J. Methotrexate for ankylosing spondylitis. *Cochrane Database Syst Rev*. 2006;(4):CD004524.

17. Chen J, Liu C. Is sulfasalazine effective in ankylosing spondylitis? A systematic review of randomized controlled trials. *J Rheumatol*. 2006;33(4):722–731.

18. van Denderen JC, van der Paardt M, Nurmohamed MT, de Ryck YM, Dijkmans BA, van der Horst-Bruinsma IE. Double-blind, randomised, placebo controlled study of leflunomide in the treatment of active ankylosing spondylitis. *Ann Rheum Dis*. 2005;64(12):1761–1764.

19. Günaydin I, Pereira PL, Daikeler T, et al. Magnetic resonance imaging-guided corticosteroid injection of the sacroiliac joints in patients with therapy-resistant spondyloarthropathy: a pilot study. *J Rheumatol*. 2000;27(2):424–428.

20. Maugars Y, Mathis C, Berthelot JM, Charlier C, Prost A. Assessment of the efficacy of sacroiliac corticosteroid injections in spondylarthropathies: a double-blind study. *Br J Rheumatol*. 1996;35(8):767–770.

21. Braun J, Bollow M, Seyrekbasan F, et al. Computed tomography-guided corticosteroid injection of the sacroiliac joint in patients with spondyloarthropathy

with sacroiliitis: clinical outcome and follow-up by dynamic magnetic resonance imaging. *J Rheumatol.* 1996;23(4):659–664.

22. Huang F, Gu J, Zhao W, Zhu J, Zhang J, Yu DT. One-year open-label trial of thalidomide in ankylosing spondylitis. *Arthritis Rheum.* 2002;47:249–254.

23. Maksymowych WP, Jhangri GS, Fitzgerald AA, et al. A six-month randomized, controlled, double-blind, dose-response comparison of intravenous pamidronate (60 mg versus 10 mg) in the treatment of nonsteroidal antiinflammatory drug-refractory ankylosing spondylitis. *Arthritis Rheum.* 2002;46(3):766–773.

24. Khan MA, Sieper J. Reactive arthritis. In Koopman WJ, Moreland LW, eds. *Arthritis and Allied Conditions*, 15th ed. Philadelphia: Lippincott Williams & Wilkins; 2004:1335–1355.

Chapter 12

The new treatment: Remarkable efficacy of TNF-α antagonists

TNF-α inhibitors have transformed the management of AS and related SpA.[1-10] Patients who do not respond to conventional therapies can now be offered treatment with these agents. Etanercept (Enbrel), infliximab (Remicade), and adalimumab (Humira) are now approved by the U.S. Food and Drug Administration (FDA) for the treatment of AS and PsA, in addition to RA and psoriasis. (A fourth TNF-α antagonist, golimumab, is expected to be approved by the FDA by time this book is published). These TNF-α inhibitors are highly and equally effective as monotherapy (without the need for concomitant methotrexate [MTX]) for treating musculoskeletal manifestations in patients with active AS unresponsive to conventional therapy. They lead to rapid and remarkable improvement in the symptoms and signs, including back pain and stiffness, peripheral arthritis, enthesitis, and dactylitis, and they have maintained long-term effectiveness.[11-16] Clinical improvement is accompanied by a significant decrease in inflammation, as evidenced by a dramatic reduction in CRP and ESR. The improvement also may be shown on MRI, but it is too early to say whether these medications will slow or prevent progressive bony ankylosis.[17-19]

These biologics are also very effective in treating PsA, as well as the cutaneous and nail lesions of psoriasis. A few patients with ReA and undifferentiated SpA that are refractory to traditional therapies have been treated with TNF-α inhibitors and have also shown good response. Infliximab and adalimumab (monoclonal antibodies) are effective in managing IBD, but etanercept (a receptor-fusion protein) lacks such an effect. Infliximab is FDA approved for treating both ulcerative colitis and Crohn's disease, while adalimumab is approved for treating Crohn's disease. The monoclonals may also be more effective in preventing recurrences of acute anterior uveitis.[20,21]

Etanercept (50 mg once weekly or 25 mg twice weekly as a subcutaneous injection) has been shown to be tolerable and efficacious in decreasing symptoms and signs of active AS, as well as improving function, spine mobility, and quality of life. Infliximab (5 mg/kg by intravenous infusion at weeks 0, 2, and 6 and subsequently every 6 weeks) has shown consistent efficacy in controlling the symptoms and signs of AS, as well as improving productivity and reducing workday loss. Continuous treatment of AS with infliximab is more efficacious than on-demand treatment, and the addition of MTX to infliximab provides no significant benefit.[6]

The ASAS response criteria have been used to demonstrate sustained, long-term efficacy of all three TNF antagonists. For example, all patients with AS in a multicenter, open-label extension of a previous 24-week, double-blind, randomized-controlled study of etanercept, who subsequently enrolled in the open-label extension study (n = 257), were followed for up to 192 weeks during the open-label portion of the study (Fig. 12.1).[5] Not shown in the figure are the ASAS20 and ASAS40 responses when calculated for the subjects who had at least one post-dose assessment, using last observation carried forward (LOCF) for missing data imputation. These responses were 67% for ASAS20 and 49% for ASAS40.

The ASAS response criteria were also used to assess the long-term efficacy of infliximab over 5 years in 69 patients with active AS.[7] After completing the 3-month, placebo-controlled, randomized phase of the study, 65 of the 69 patients entered an open-label study and received intravenous infliximab (5 mg/kg every 6 weeks). Completer analysis of all 35 patients who completed the entire 5-year period is shown in Figure 12.2A. There were significant and sustained reductions (indicating clinical improvement) in BASDAI, BASFI, and BASMI scores and also significant improvement in the percentage of AS patients who achieved ASAS40 and ASAS5/6 responses during 5 years of infliximab treatment in the open-label portion of the study. At 5 years, ASAS40 and -5/6 response rates were 63.4% and 68.3%, respectively, and 65% showed at least 50% reduction in the BASDAI score (BASDAI 50 response) (Fig 12.2B). Adalimumab was the last of the three TNF antagonists to gain FDA approval for the treatment of AS; the therapeutic dosage is 40 mg every other week. It has been shown to be safe and efficacious in patients with active AS: the percentages of patients who achieved an ASAS20 and an ASAS5/6 response were equal to the other two TNF antagonists.[8]

Adalimumab, like the other TNF antagonists, significantly reduced both spinal and SI joint inflammation in patients with active AS after 12 weeks of treatment, and these improvements were maintained for up to 52 weeks.[9]

A recent study has shown the clinical efficacy of adalimumab in patients with early axial SpA, before the occurrence of radiographically confirmed sacroiliitis. In this 52-week, randomized, controlled trial of 46 patients with NSAID-refractory pre-radiographic axial SpA,[22] patients were randomized to placebo (n = 24) or adalimumab (n = 22) for 12 weeks, followed by an open-label extension for up to 52 weeks (Fig. 12.3). After 12 weeks, ASAS40 responses and ASAS partial remissions were achieved in 54.5% and 22.7%, respectively, of the adalimumab-treated patients, compared with 12.5% and 0% of the placebo-treated patients (p = 0.004 and p = 0.019, respectively). At 52 weeks, ASAS40 responses and ASAS partial remissions were sustained in patients continually treated with adalimumab throughout the study (45.5% and 18.2%, respectively). Patients who switched from placebo to adalimumab at 12 weeks during the open-label extension showed significant improvements in ASAS40 and ASAS partial

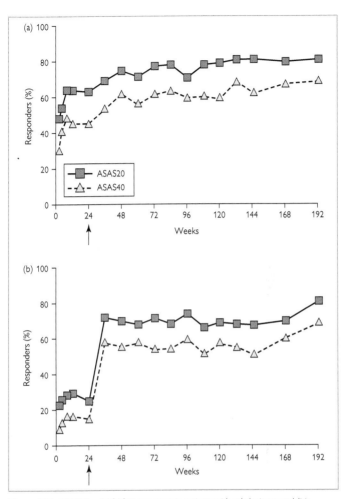

Figure 12.1 ASAS20 and ASAS40 responses in patients with ankylosing spondylitis treated with etanercept. (A) Results in patients treated with etanercept. (B) Results in patients treated with placebo for the first 24 weeks and then switched to etanercept. After 192 weeks of etanercept exposure, the ASAS20 response was 81% and the ASAS40 response was 69% in the completer analysis (for all patients remaining in the trial at that time). Not shown in this figure are the ASAS20 and ASAS40 responses when calculated for the subjects who had at least one post-dose assessment, using LOCF (Last Observation Carried Forward) for missing data imputation. These responses were 67% for ASAS20 and 49% for ASAS40. Reprinted, with permission from BMJ Publishing Ltd., from Davis JC Jr, van Der Heijde D, Braun J, et al. Efficacy and safety of up to 192 weeks of etanercept therapy in patients with ankylosing spondylitis. *Ann Rheum Dis.* 2008;67:346–352.

responses (50.0% and 37.5%, respectively; p = 0.004 and p = 0.002). The fact that a substantial percentage of patients achieved partial remission suggests that TNF antagonists may be even more effective in early forms of axial SpA.

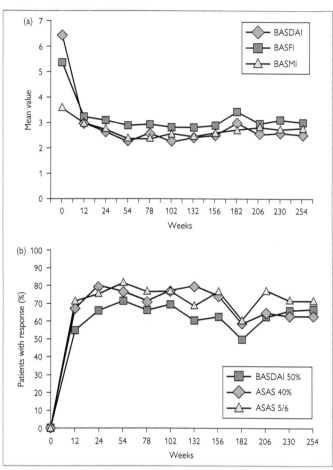

Figure 12.2 Long-term efficacy of infliximab in treating patients with ankylosing spondylitis (completer analysis of all 35 patients who completed the entire 5-year study period). (A) There were significant and sustained reductions (indicating clinical improvement) in BASDAI, BASFI, and BASMI. (B) There were also significant and sustained improvements as judged by the percentage of patients achieving ASAS40 or ASAS5/6 responses, or at least 50% reduction in BASDAI score. Reprinted, with permission from BMJ Publishing, Ltd., from Braun J, Baraliakos X, Listing J, et al. Persistent clinical efficacy and safety of anti-tumour necrosis factor alpha therapy with infliximab in patients with ankylosing spondylitis over 5 years: evidence for different types of response. *Ann Rheum Dis.* 2008;67(3):340–345.

Improvements in spinal inflammation observed on MRI

A characteristic feature of AS is the progression of axial inflammation from the sacroiliac joints to the intervertebral discs, facet joints, and ligamentous

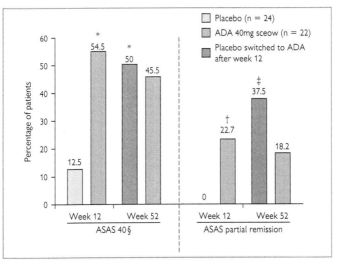

Figure 12.3 Results of adalimumab in pre-radiographic axial undifferentiated spondyloarthropathy (early ankylosing spondylitis without x-ray defined sacroiliitis). Forty-six patients completed the12-week randomly controlled trial, and 38 completed the 52-week open-label extension phase of the study. At week 12, 54.5% of patients receiving adalimumab showed ASAS40 response versus 12.5% on placebo (p = 0.004). After switching to adalimumab, those patients who were initially on placebo also showed a similar degree of efficacy. At week 52, the efficacy was maintained in all patients. The bars indicate the percentage of patients who achieved ASAS40 and ASAS partial-remission responses at 12 weeks and at 52 weeks. Young age and an elevated CRP were the best predictors of the ASAS40 response (not shown in this figure). Reprinted, with permission from John Wiley and Sons, Inc., from Haibel H, Rudwaleit M, Amtenbrink A, et al. Efficacy of adalimumab in the treatment of preradiographic axial spondyloarthritis: 52-week results of a randomized controlled trial and open-label extension. *Arthritis Rheum.* 2008;58(7):1981–1991.

structures of the spine. This progression is typically assessed in clinical practice using plane radiography; however, scoring methods to measure radiographic structural change have shown poor sensitivity to change. MRI of the spine in patients with AS has shown abnormalities of the spine before the development of typical features on plane radiographs.[23–25]

Treatment with TNF-α inhibitors is associated with a decrease in spinal inflammation as detected by MRI; it was persistently reduced in all patients constantly treated with infliximab, but it was not eradicated.[14–18] Disease activity parameters do not directly correlate with MRI, but both point in the same direction, indicating that both the disease activity parameters and the MRI response may be useful for defining response to anti-TNF therapy. Treatment with the TNF antagonists increases bone density in patients with AS.[26,27]

Halting or reducing radiographic progression in AS

Halting or reducing radiographic progression of disease is essential in the management of AS; this has already been shown when patients with RA and PsA were treated with TNF antagonists. TNF antagonists do target sites of active inflammation, but we need to know whether they also directly inhibit osteoproliferation (see Chapter 4).

The effect of infliximab on radiographic structural changes was evaluated over a period of 4 years in 33 patients with AS using the modified Stoke ankylosing spondylitis spine score (mSASSS); in this scoring system, definite radiographic progression is defined as a change in mSASSS from 0 (no damage) or 1 (suspicious damage) to more than 2 (syndesmophytes or ankylosis). Radiographs of the cervical and lumbar spine were obtained at baseline and after 2 and 4 years of infliximab treatment and scored in a concealed time order. The mean mSASSS score changed from 11.6 at baseline to 12.5 at 2 years and 13.2 at 4 years ($p < 0.05$ versus baseline).[17] Definite radiographic progression was observed in 30.3% of patients between baseline and 4 years, but the change in the mean mSASSS score (reflecting the degree of definite radiographic progression) observed with infliximab over 4 years was less pronounced compared to published data from a historical Outcome Assessments in Ankylosing Spondylitis International Study (OASIS) cohort not treated with TNF antagonists (1.6 versus 4.4). However, this published OASIS cohort (treated with conventional therapy [i.e., NSAIDs, DMARDs, corticosteroids, and/or analgesics]) was from earlier years and was unmatched, and therefore was not an ideal control group for comparison.

Inhibition of osteoproliferation did not occur in patients with AS during a 2-year treatment period with etanercept, even though there was resolution of bone edema on MRI, which reflects the presence of osteitis/enthesitis.[18,28,29] There is a need to study a larger number of AS patients with early disease and to treat them for a longer period to establish whether TNF antagonists do or do not inhibit syndesmophyte formation. A better scoring method is also needed to assess structural damage, because the mSASSS method used in this study focuses heavily on the formation of syndesmophytes and the occurrence of ankylosis (osteoproliferation), while erosive changes (osteolysis) have a minor influence on the total score. In the meantime, AS patients taking TNF antagonists should not taper off their NSAIDs, because there is evidence that NSAIDs do seem to inhibit osteoproliferation.[30]

Uveitis

Acute anterior uveitis is an important extraarticular manifestation of AS. An analysis of four placebo-controlled studies with anti-TNF agents in AS (two with etanercept and two with infliximab) and three open-label studies showed that the patients treated with anti-TNF agents had a significant decrease in mean frequency of flares of anterior uveitis compared to the placebo group.[21] The monoclonal TNF antagonists infliximab and adalimumab are more effective than etanercept in preventing flares of uveitis in patients with AS and related SpA.[21,22,31] Paradoxically, TNF antagonists also seem to induce uveitis in some patients, probably more often after treatment with etanercpt.[31,32]

CHAPTER 12 TNF-α antagonists

Guidelines for the use of TNF-α antagonists for AS

The ASAS has developed a consensus statement for the use of TNF-α inhibitors for AS (Table 12.1).[10] For initiation of such treatment, there should be a diagnosis of definite AS (normally based on modified New York criteria). The disease must be active for at least 4 weeks, as determined by a BASDAI of at least 4 on a 0-to-10 scale. Initiation of such treatment requires distinguishing symptoms that reflect active disease from symptoms of a mechanical or psychological nature ("expert opinion" based on additional supportive clinical findings) and presence of refractory disease based on failure of at least two NSAIDs during a 3-month period (unless there is intolerance, toxicity, or contraindications to their use), failure of intraarticular corticosteroids (if indicated), and failure of sulfasalazine in patients with predominantly peripheral arthritis. Moreover, one needs to apply the usual precautions and contraindications for biological treatment.

Treatment must be continued on a long-term basis to maintain disease control. When one TNF-α inhibitor has not succeeded or adverse effects develop that are not related to the TNF-α inhibitors as a class, switching to another agent may be indicated.[4,33] Both the BASDAI and the ASAS core set for clinical practice (see Chapter 10) should be followed for monitoring the treatment with TNF-α inhibitors. Response is defined as improvement of at least 50% or 2 units (on a 0-to-10 scale) of the BASDAI score. Discontinuation of anti-TNF treatment should be considered if the patient fails to respond after 12 weeks of treatment.[10]

Possible safety issues with TNF antagonists and contraindications are listed in Tables 12.2 and 12.3.[1,34,35] Possible adverse effects include allergic reactions, especially with intravenous infliximab administration, injection site reactions (with subcutaneous administration of etanercept and adalimumab), and an increased risk of infections (including opportunistic infections, such as reactivation or occurrence of tuberculosis or histoplasmosis, and also activation of some of the preexisting viral infections [e.g., hepatitis B virus]). All patients should receive pneumococcal and yearly influenza vaccinations, ideally before starting TNF antagonist therapy.

A PPD skin test is recommended to screen for prior exposure to *Mycobacterium tuberculosis*, and patients showing a positive skin reaction (induration of 5 mm or more) need to be treated before starting TNF antagonist therapy.[35] Interferon-γ-based testing may also be needed in some patients as a part of the pretreatment workup if detecting latent TB infection is crucial, but neither test can differentiate active from latent TB.[36] Physicians should monitor patients receiving TNF-α antagonists for signs

Table 12.1 ASAS consensus statement on use of TNF antagonists in patients with AS

Diagnosis:

A diagnosis of definitive AS, normally fulfilling modified New York criteria for definitive AS

Disease activity:

Presence of active disease for at least 4 weeks as defined by both

• Sustained BASDAI >4 and

• An expert opinion based on clinical features, acute phase reactants, and imaging modalities

Previous treatment:

• All patients should have had adequate therapeutic trials of at least two NSAIDs for at least 3 months at maximum recommended or tolerated anti-inflammatory dose, unless contraindicated or treatment was withdrawn because of intolerance, toxicity, or contraindications.

• Patients with pure axial manifestations do not have to take DMARDs before anti-TNF treatment can be started.

• Patients with symptomatic peripheral arthritis should have an insufficient response to at least one local corticosteroid injection if appropriate.

• Patients with (primarily) persistent peripheral arthritis must have had a therapeutic trial of sulfasalazine.

• Patients with (primarily) symptomatic enthesitis must have failed appropriate local treatment.

Dosing:

Etanercept 50 mg subcutaneously once a week

Infliximab 5 mg/kg IV every 6 to 8 weeks

Adalimumab 40 mg subcutaneously every other week

Responder criteria:

50% improvement of BASDAI or absolute change of 2 on 0 cm to 10 cm scale and "expert" opinion that treatment should be continued (based on clinical features, acute phase reactants, and imaging modalities)

Time of evaluation:

Between 6 and 12 weeks

Precautions:

Usual precautions and contraindications for biological therapy

Tuberculosis precautions:

Use country-specific guidelines.

and symptoms of active TB (including patients who tested negative for latent TB infection) or other opportunistic infections. Treatment of latent TB should be initiated prior to therapy with a TNF-α antagonist. All patients with evidence of latent TB infection, after active TB has been excluded, should be treated with isoniazid (INH) 300 mg daily for 9 months, with supplemental vitamin B_6 (50 mg daily in patients with a predisposition for peripheral neuropathy). Patients from areas with high rates of INH-resistant TB need treatment with rifampin, and infectious disease consultation should be considered. Patients exposed to multidrug-resistant TB need infectious disease consultation; potential therapies may include pyrazinamide along with either ethambutol or fluoroquinolone for 6 to 12 months.[35]

Other rare adverse effects of TNF antagonists include demyelinating disease, lupus-like syndromes, exacerbation of congestive heart failure, and malignancy (Table 12.2).[34] TNF inhibitors are considered category B drugs in pregnancy and should be avoided during pregnancy or lactation. Other possible contraindications are listed in Table 12.3.

Summary

- TNF antagonists are remarkably effective in AS, even more so than in RA. They need to be used on a long-term basis to maintain disease control.
- There is no need to use MTX prior to or with anti-TNF therapy to manage AS.
- Traditional DMARDs (including MTX) do not work in axial disease of AS.

Table 12.2 Possible safety issues with TNF antagonists

Infections: Serious infections, opportunistic infections, and preexisting viral infections (such as hepatitis B virus)
Reaction to infusion and local injection
Autoantibodies, antichimeric antibodies, and lupus-like syndrome
Malignancies: Lymphoma, skin cancers, solid organ cancers
Demyelinating conditions
Congestive heart failure
Pregnancy and lactation

Table 12.3 Possible contraindications for treatment with TNF antagonists

Patients with active infection or at high risk of infection, including:
1. Septic arthritis of a native joint within the past 12 months
2. Sepsis of a prosthetic joint within the past 12 months (or indefinitely if the prosthesis remains in situ)
3. Chronic leg ulcers
4. Indwelling urinary catheter
5. Persistent or recurrent chest infections
History of multiple sclerosis or lupus
Malignancy or premalignancy states (but excluding basal cell carcinoma and malignancies diagnosed and treated more than 10 years previously [indicating high probability of total cure])
Women who are pregnant or breastfeeding

- All three TNF antagonists are remarkably effective for musculoskeletal features. The response is better in earlier stages of disease. They are also effective in axial undifferentiated SpA.
- Treatment with TNF inhibitors results in substantial improvements in signs and symptoms of axial and peripheral arthritis as well as enthesitis, dactylitis, uveitis, and skin and bowel disease.
- There are differences between the monoclonal antibodies (infliximab and adalimumab) and etanercept with regard to their extraarticular efficacy. For example, etanercept is not effective in controlling Crohn's disease and ulcerative colitis.
- Approved dosages are as follows:
  - Infliximab: 5 mg/kg (induction regimen weeks 0, 2, 6 and then every 6 weeks as a maintenance dose)
  - Etanercept: 50 mg subcutaneously each week
  - Adalimumab: 40 mg subcutaneously every other week

Concluding remarks

Physical functioning can be markedly affected by AS, leading to limitations in the patient's ability to work. NSAIDs and physical therapy are the traditional first-line treatments for AS, but many patients fail to respond adequately to these interventions. MTX and other conventional DMARDs are not effective as second-line treatments for managing the axial manifestations of AS. The demonstrated efficacy of TNF antagonists in patients with AS who show an inadequate response to conventional therapy has enabled physicians to manage treatment more effectively. TNF antagonists are highly effective in AS in alleviating pain and reducing clinical disease activity, both axial and peripheral arthritis, reducing spinal and sacroiliac joint inflammation as visualized on MRI, alleviating extraarticular manifestations, improving quality of life, and maintaining long-term efficacy out to 5 years. The response is greater in patients with earlier disease and less damage. The untoward effects of anti-TNF therapy in AS do not appear to be much different from those in RA and PsA. It is important to screen for latent TB before starting this therapy.

Many AS patients who meet the criteria for anti-TNF treatment according to published guidelines do not receive this treatment for one reason or another (including cost and possible side effects). This therapy is also very effective in patients with pre-radiographic AS (axial undifferentiated spondyloarthritis) and could be extended to this early phase of the disease in hopes of slowing, if not preventing, radiologic progression and ankylosis.

Additional TNF antagonists (e.g., golimumab and certolizumab pegol) are in various stages of clinical studies and are expected to be approved by the FDA and the European Medicines Agency (European equivalent of FDA) in the near future for the treatment of AS and related SpA. Certolizumab (Cimzia) has just been approved by the FDA for the treatment of Crohn's disease.

References

1. Ackermann C, Kavanaugh A. Tumor necrosis factor as a therapeutic target of rheumatologic disease. *Expert Opin Ther Targets*. 2007;11(11):1369–1384.

2. McLeod C, Bagust A, Boland A, et al. Adalimumab, etanercept and infliximab for the treatment of ankylosing spondylitis: a systematic review and economic evaluation. *Health Technol Assess*. 2007;11(28):1–158.

3. Heiberg MS, Koldingsnes W, Mikkelsen K, et al. The comparative one-year performance of anti-tumor necrosis factor alpha drugs in patients with rheumatoid arthritis, psoriatic arthritis, and ankylosing spondylitis: results from a longitudinal, observational, multicenter study. *Arthritis Rheum*. 2008;59(2):234–240.

4. Coates LC, Cawkwell LS, Ng NW, et al. Real-life experience confirms sustained response to long-term biologics and switching in ankylosing spondylitis. *Rheumatology (Oxford)*. 2008;47(6):897–900.

5. Davis JC Jr, van Der Heijde D, Braun J, et al. Efficacy and safety of up to 192 weeks of etanercept therapy in patients with ankylosing spondylitis. *Ann Rheum Dis*. 2008;67:346–352.

6. Breban M, Ravaud P, Claudepierre P, et al. Maintenance of infliximab treatment in ankylosing spondylitis: results of a one-year randomized controlled trial comparing systematic versus on-demand treatment. *Arthritis Rheum*. 2007;58(1):88–97.

7. Braun J, Baraliakos X, Listing J, et al. Persistent clinical efficacy and safety of anti-tumour necrosis factor alpha therapy with infliximab in patients with ankylosing spondylitis over 5 years: evidence for different types of response. *Ann Rheum Dis*. 2008;67(3):340–345.

8. van der Heijde D, Kivitz A, Schiff MH, et al. Efficacy and safety of adalimumab in patients with ankylosing spondylitis: results of a multicenter, randomized, double-blind, placebo-controlled trial. *Arthritis Rheum*. 2006;54(7):2136–2146.

9. Lambert RG, Salonen D, Rahman P. Adalimumab significantly reduces both spinal and sacroiliac joint inflammation in patients with ankylosing spondylitis: a multicenter, randomized, double-blind, placebo-controlled study. *Arthritis Rheum*. 2007;56(12):4005–4014.

10. Braun J, Davis J, Dougados M, Sieper J, vaan der Linden S, van der Heijde D, ASAS Working Group. First update of the international ASAS consensus statement for the use of anti-TNF agents in patients with ankylosing spondylitis. *Ann Rheum Dis*. 2006;65(3):316–320.

11. van der Heijde D, Han C, DeVlam K, et al. Infliximab improves productivity and reduces workday loss in patients with ankylosing spondylitis: results from a randomized, placebo-controlled trial. *Arthritis Rheum*. 2006;55(4):569–574.

12. Braun J, McHugh N, Singh A, Wajdula JS, Sato R. Improvement in patient-reported outcomes for patients with ankylosing spondylitis treated with etanercept 50 mg once-weekly and 25 mg twice-weekly. *Rheumatology (Oxford)*. 2007;46(6):999–1004.

13. Davis JC Jr, Revicki D, van der Heijde DM, et al. Health-related quality of life outcomes in patients with active ankylosing spondylitis treated with adalimumab: results from a randomized controlled study. *Arthritis Rheum*. 2007;57(6):1050–1057.

14. Braun J, Landewe R, Hermann KG, et al. Major reduction in spinal inflammation in patients with ankylosing spondylitis after treatment with infliximab: results of a multicenter, randomized, double-blind, placebo-controlled magnetic resonance imaging study. *Arthritis Rheum*. 2006;54(5):1646–1652.

15. Baraliakos X, Davis J, Tsuji W, Braun J. Magnetic resonance imaging examinations of the spine in patients with ankylosing spondylitis before and after therapy with the tumor necrosis factor alpha receptor fusion protein etanercept. *Arthritis Rheum.* 2005;52(4):1216–1223.

16. Haibel H, Rudwaleit M, Brandt HC, et al. Adalimumab reduces spinal symptoms in active ankylosing spondylitis: clinical and magnetic resonance imaging results of a fifty-two-week open-label trial. *Arthritis Rheum.* 2006;54(2):678–681.

17. Baraliakos X, Listing J, Brandt J, et al. Radiographic progression in patients with ankylosing spondylitis after 4 yrs of treatment with the anti-TNF-alpha antibody infliximab. *Rheumatology (Oxford).* 2007;46(9):1450–1453.

18. van der Heijde D, Landewé R, Einstein S, et al. Radiographic progression of ankylosing spondylitis after up to two years of treatment with etanercept. *Arthritis Rheum.* 2008;58(5):1324–1331.

19. Sieper J, Appel H, Braun J, Rudwaleit M. Critical appraisal of assessment of structural damage in ankylosing spondylitis: implications for treatment outcomes. *Arthritis Rheum.* 2008;58(3):649–656.

20. Braun J, Baraliakos X, Listing J, Sieper J. Decreased incidence of anterior uveitis in patients with ankylosing spondylitis treated with the anti-tumor necrosis factor agents infliximab and etanercept. *Arthritis Rheum.* 2005;52(8):2447–2451.

21. Guignard S, Gossec L, Salliot C, et al. Efficacy of tumour necrosis factor blockers in reducing uveitis flares in patients with spondylarthropathy: a retrospective study. *Ann Rheum Dis.* 2006;65(12):1631–1634.

22. Haibel H, Rudwaleit M, Amtenbrink A, et al. Efficacy of adalimumab in the treatment of preradiographic axial spondyloarthritis: 52-week results of a randomized controlled trial and open-label extension. *Arthritis Rheum.* 2007;56(9 suppl): Abstract 753.

23. Weber U, Pfirrmann CWA, Kissling RO, MacKenzie CR, Khan MA. Early spondyloarthritis in HLA-B27 positive monozygotic twin pair: a highly concordant onset, sites of involvement, and disease course. *J Rheumatol.* 2008;35(7):1464–1466.

24. Weber U, Pfirrmann CW, Kissling RO, Hodler J, Zanetti M. Whole-body MR imaging in ankylosing spondylitis: a descriptive pilot study in patients with suspected early and active confirmed ankylosing spondylitis. *BMC Musculoskelet Disord.* 2007;8:20.

25. Weber U, Pfirrmann CWA, Khan MA. Ankylosing spondylitis: update on imaging and therapy. *Intl J Adv Rheumatol.* 2007;5:2–7.

26. Briot K, Gossec L, Kolta S, Dougados M, Roux C. Prospective assessment of body weight, body composition, and bone density changes in patients with spondyloarthropathy receiving anti-tumor necrosis factor-alpha treatment. *J Rheumatol.* 2008;35(5):855–861.

27. Demis E, Roux C, Breban M, Dougados M. Infliximab in spondylarthropathy—influence on bone density. *Clin Exp Rheumatol.* 2002;20:S185–186.

28. Schett G, Landewe R, van der Heijde D. Tumour necrosis factor blockers and structural remodelling in ankylosing spondylitis: what is reality and what is fiction? *Ann Rheum Dis.* 2007;66(6):709–711.

29. van der Heijde D, Landewe R, van der Linden S. How should treatment effect on spinal radiographic progression in patients with ankylosing spondylitis be measured? *Arthritis Rheum.* 2005;52(7):1979–1985.

30. Wanders A, Heijde D, Landewé R, et al. Nonsteroidal antiinflammatory drugs reduce radiographic progression in patients with ankylosing spondylitis: a randomized clinical trial. *Arthritis Rheum.* 2005;52(6):1756–1765.

31. Lim LL, Fraunfelder FW, Rosenbaum JT. Do tumor necrosis factor inhibitors cause uveitis? A registry-based study. *Arthritis Rheum*. 2007;56(10):3248–3252.

32. Coates LC, McGonagle DG, Bennett AN, Emery P, Marzo-Oetega H. Uveitis and tumor necrosis factor blockade in ankylosing spondylitis. *Ann Rheum Dis*. 2008;67:729–730.

33. Conti F, Ceccarelli F, Marocchi E, et al. Switching TNF-alpha antagonists in patients with ankylosing spondylitis and psoriatic arthritis: an observational study over a five-year period. *Ann Rheum Dis*. 2007;66(10):1393–1397.

34. Lee SJ, Kavanaugh A. Biologic agents in rheumatology: safety considerations. *Rheum Dis Clin North Am*. 2006;32(Suppl 1):3–10.

35. Ellerin T, Rubin RH, Weinblatt ME. Infections and anti-tumor necrosis factor alpha therapy. *Arthritis Rheum*. 2003;48(11):3013–3022.

36. Bergeron A, Herrmann J-L. Screening for tuberculosis before TNFa antagonist initiation: Are current methods good enough? *Joint Bone Spine*. 2008;75:112–115.

Chapter 13

Other aspects of disease management

Patients with AS should be followed on a regular basis to monitor disease activity, response to treatment, and medication side effects, even if their illness seems to be inactive.[1-3] The frequency of monitoring should be based on the clinical presentation and the drug therapy being used. Monitoring should comprise symptoms and signs, laboratory testing, and imaging studies. Specific skeletal elements to be monitored include duration of morning stiffness, severity of pain, mobility of the lumbar and cervical spine, chest expansion, and clinical evidence of enthesitis and changes in joint inflammation as well as range of motion. Measures to evaluate disease activity, such as BASDAI, BASMI, BASFI, and HAQ, may be used to monitor response to therapy.

CRP and ESR are not as useful as in patients with RA. Other laboratory tests to be monitored include complete blood count, renal function, and liver function tests to identify any therapy-related adverse effects. Radiographic monitoring of axial involvement once every 2 years is usually sufficient but can be done more frequently in select patients. Radiographs, however, are not sensitive for changes over less than 1 year. Lateral cervical and lumbar spine films are usually sufficient, but radiographs of the thoracic spine are sometimes needed, especially when a fracture is suspected.

Patient education

Health education for self-management in patients with chronic arthritis produces sustained health benefits and reduces health-care costs. Patients should be educated about the nature of their illness and their prognosis and should be encouraged to assume a central role in managing their illness.[4] Self-help programs in patients with arthritis facilitate adherence to drug regimens, decrease pain, and increase knowledge. Smoking cessation should be urged because smokers have more severe illness and an increased incidence of respiratory complications, in addition to the numerous other adverse effects of smoking. The role of pharmacological and nonpharmacological therapies should be clearly explained to patients, and they should be given information about relevant associations, books, pamphlets, videos, and audiotapes.[4]

Some useful Web sites include the following:

http://www.spondylitis.org
http://www.asif.rheumanet.org

http://www.arthritis.org
http://patients.uptodate.com

Patients should be advised to sleep on a firm mattress without a pillow, if possible, or with a thin pillow or a pillow that is suitably contoured to maintain neck extension and prevent spinal deformities from developing. They should be encouraged to walk erectly, keeping the spine as straight as possible while maintaining normal, reciprocal arm swing and rotational movements of the lower spine and pelvis during walking. Stooped postures such as slouching in chairs or leaning over a desk for prolonged periods should be avoided; adjustable swivel chairs with lumbar support and elevated and inclined writing surfaces may be helpful. Patients should maintain hip extension, for example by lying prone for a 15-minute period daily. Crossing roads should be done with caution due to impaired neck mobility.

Restrictions/disability-related issues

Problems in performing activities of daily living should be identified and solutions should be sought to compensate for loss of motion and to improve functional capacity. Common functional difficulties include dressing, body transfers, lifting and carrying, and endurance. Patients should be advised to make helpful home and workplace modifications. They should avoid prolonged immobility at home or at work and should change position frequently and take breaks for body stretching.

Postural changes that occur because the center of mass of the trunk is displaced can affect balance and pose safety concerns. It is important to take steps to prevent falls, such as avoiding loose carpets and installing night lights. Bathrooms should have nonslippery floors and should be equipped with features such as railings, grab bars, and safety mats.

Patients with advanced disease may need assistive devices. These devices include walking aids if the patient has lower extremity joint problems, adjustable swivel chairs with lumbar support, elevated and inclined writing surfaces, and long-handled devices for dressing and for reaching or picking up objects. Back splints, braces, and corsets are not helpful and should be avoided.

Driving

Many AS patients with a painful and stiff spine have difficulty driving a long distance and find it useful to stop after an hour or two to get out of the car, stretch the back, and walk around for a few minutes. Patients must always wear seat belts and use proper head, neck, and back support. It is better to avoid bucket seats. Patients should use headrests (head restraints) so that sudden slowing or stopping does not jerk the spine, including the neck; the stiff neck of an AS patient is more vulnerable to injury than a normal neck. The top of the headrest should be level with the top of the driver's head and as close to the back of the head as possible.

Decreased range of motion of the cervical spine makes driving a real challenge. The use of wide-angled mirrors increases the driver's peripheral vision, making driving easier and safer. Patients may find it difficult to back the car into the garage and other tight parking spaces because they cannot turn their neck to look behind them. Special mirrors fitted onto the car can help; the patient should take a few practice sessions backing up the car in an open area to become comfortable using these mirrors. Disabled driver parking permits may be appropriate for patients who cannot walk very far, but this is usually not a problem for most patients with AS.

"Medical Alert" card

It is useful for patients with AS to carry a "Medical Alert" card that contains concise information about them. The card should identify the degree of forward bending of the neck and the appropriate precautions that need to be taken in case of an emergency. A proposed version of such a card is shown in Box 13.1.

Box 13.1 Medical alert card for patients with AS, especially those with advanced disease

My name is _____.

I suffer from **ankylosing spondylitis,** a form of arthritis that has caused a severe limitation of motion of my back and neck.

My home and/or work phone: _____

In emergency call: _____   Cell phone: _____

My Physician/Hospital name/phone: _____

My Physician/Hospital Fax/e-mail: _____

I am allergic to: _____

My daily medications:

_____

My other illnesses (besides ankylosing spondylitis):

_____
_____

CAUTION: My whole spine is fused (rigid), including my neck.

I am prone to easily fracturing my neck or my back, and it can happen even after a trivial injury. Spinal fracture, if it is unstable or is not properly immobilized, can lead to paralysis or death.

Be careful and avoid any movement of my neck and back while lifting me onto a stretcher or an examining table, and during any procedure, such as radiography (x-rays) or insertion of a tube in the windpipe (trachea) for breathing or general anesthesia. My rib cage is also fused, and therefore I have very limited chest expansion. I breathe mainly by using my diaphragm.

Before any x-ray or other imaging studies (MRI or CT), my fused (rigid) and forwardly stooped neck or any part of my spine **MUST** be kept in its usual alignment (during conventional immobilization by emergency services before radiographic or surgical procedures).

My neck is forwardly stooped by roughly _____ degrees.

CAUTION: Excessive straightening of my neck or spine into a "normal" position can make a stable fracture unstable and may result in paralysis or death. Plain x-rays of the neck and back may not detect the fracture, and it may require MRI or CT.

For additional information on my disease, suitable Web sites include www.spondylitis.org, www.asif.rheumanet.org, and www.hlab27.com.

Referrals/consultations

In cases of acute anterior uveitis, ophthalmological evaluation is urgently needed. For other extraskeletal complications, referral to a cardiologist, pulmonologist, or other specialist may be needed. Depression is not uncommon in patients with any chronic painful illness that impairs quality of life, and this includes AS. Depression is a treatable disease that has many underlying causes, and some individuals are genetically prone to depression.

Role of surgery

Total hip replacement is indicated in patients with advanced hip involvement who have severe pain or functional disability. There is no significant increase in the incidence of heterotopic bone formation or ankylosis following this surgery, although some surgeons may use NSAIDs for 7 to 10 days, starting from the day of surgery. Similarly, the involvement of other joints, especially the knee, may require joint replacement in advanced cases. Other elective surgeries that might be indicated include corrective spinal wedge osteotomy to correct severe kyphosis and uncompensated loss of horizontal vision, and spinal fusion procedures for instability, including atlantoaxial subluxation, pseudarthrosis, and fracture. Spinal pseudarthrosis should be differentiated from indolent infections.

Any new-onset neck or back pain in a patient with AS should be evaluated carefully for a spinal fracture or instability, even in the absence of obvious physical trauma or after a seemingly trivial injury, because paraplegia or quadriplegia may result. The back or neck should be immobilized in its usual alignment as a precaution pending musculoskeletal imaging if fracture is suspected; excessive straightening into a "normal" position can make a stable fracture unstable and may result in paralysis or death. The radiographic findings may be normal, and MRI, CT, or bone scan results may be more helpful in confirming or excluding spinal fracture.

Heart complications may require aortic valve replacement or placement of a cardiac pacemaker. Scarring (fibrosis) and cavity (cyst) formation in the upper part (apex) of the lung is not easy to manage, and surgical resection may (rarely) be required.

In patients with AS who undergo surgery, special care must be taken to avoid pulmonary complications, which are more likely to occur in these patients because of their decreased vital capacity and restricted chest wall expansion.

Anesthesia

Lumbar spinal anesthesia by lumbar puncture may not be possible due to spinal fusion and ligament ossification, although epidural block may be possible. General anesthesia can be a challenge for both the anesthesiologist and the surgeon. The anesthesiologist may have difficulty passing a breathing tube down the trachea so that the airway can be maintained during general anesthesia. This is a potential problem in patients with a rigid spine, especially if the patient also has forward stooping of the neck and a reduced jaw-opening capacity. Some patients with extreme neck deformity may require a tracheostomy.

The patient should discuss these issues with the surgeon and should have a preoperative consultation with the anesthesiologist. The patient should not assume that all health-care providers are fully aware of the limitations due to AS. The anesthesiologist should examine the patient before surgery to identify any limitations and to allay any patient concerns. This should be done in the patient's hospital room before he or she is taken to the operating room, and before any anesthetic premedications are given that reduce the patient's alertness.

Patients with AS are also more likely to have postsurgical lung complications due to their severely restricted chest wall movement and possible intubation difficulties resulting from cervical spinal ankylosis and flexion deformity, as well as severely restricted mouth opening due to temporomandibular joint involvement or presences of atlantoaxial subluxation.

Patient concerns and questions

High-impact sports or those that involve significant abrupt movement of the spine should be strongly discouraged, especially for patients with advanced disease, because of the increased risk of spinal injury. When swimming, patients may use snorkels and masks for breathing if they have restricted motion of the neck (see Chapter 11). Badminton, walking, and cross-country (but not downhill) skiing are suitable sports. Some modifications can be made in sports that require a forward-flexed posture, such as raising bicycle handlebars. Footwear can be adjusted to reduce the impact of some activities on the spine and reduce the discomfort of heel spurs and the risk of slipping. Patients should always have a warm-up period to relieve stiffness and decrease the likelihood of injury.

Workplace needs should be evaluated, and appropriate modifications should be made. Changing position frequently and taking breaks for body stretching will improve endurance.

It is not unusual for more than one person in a family to be affected with AS or related diseases, so the physician should ask in detail about the family history. The impact of the disease on the family should be discussed with patients and possibly family members.

The patient may want to know the odds that his or her children will develop AS. Roughly 50% of the children of any HLA-B27-positive individual will inherit HLA-B27 from that parent. HLA-B27-positive children of such a patient will have an up to 1 in 5 chance of developing AS or related SpA during their lifetime. The other half of children who lack the gene carry virtually no increased risk unless other diseases that also predispose to AS (such as psoriasis or IBD) are present in the family. Thus, on average most (80%) of the B27-positive children in such families with a B27-positive parent suffering from AS are likely to remain unaffected.[4-7] Therefore, children in such families do not need to be tested for HLA-B27. Even among the 50% of children who are expected to inherit the B27 gene, most will remain unaffected during their lifetime, and at present we do not know how to prevent AS. Parents and health-care providers may unnecessarily get "HLA-B27-itis" every time the HLA-B27-positive child gets injuries and sprains. Knowing that the child has HLA-B27, the parents and health-care providers might worry unnecessarily, and symptoms unrelated to AS may be wrongly attributed to the fact that the child has inherited HLA-B27. The child may get an incorrect diagnostic label of AS, even though he or she is an unaffected individual who happens to have a normal gene called HLA-B27. Even a child who remains totally healthy may suffer indirectly in the future if the information about the HLA-B27 test result is on the medical chart and becomes available to health insurance companies or potential employers, who may misuse such information.

What if a child of a B27-positive affected parent develops symptoms (back pain and stiffness that is worsened with rest) that the parent suspects are due to early AS? The parent should raise this possibility with the child's physician, and preferably be seen by a (pediatric) rheumatologist. The physician can conduct further investigation based on the results of clinical investigation and imaging studies and, when appropriate, may use HLA-B27 typing as an aid to early diagnosis.

If the parent with primary AS does not have HLA-B27 (a 10% to 15% chance if he or she is white, and up to a 50% chance if African American), then the risk of AS among the children is virtually nonexistent, unless any of the other diseases that also predispose to AS (as mentioned above) are present in the family.

References

1. Braun J, Sieper J. Ankylosing spondylitis. *Lancet.* 2007;369(9570):1379–1390.

2. Khan MA. Ankylosing spondylitis: burden of illness, diagnosis, and effective treatment. *J Rheumatol Suppl.* 2006;78:1–33.

3. Khan MA. Update on spondyloarthropathies. *Ann Intern Med.* 2002; 136:896–907.

4. Khan MA. *Ankylosing Spondylitis: The Facts.* Oxford: Oxford University Press; 2002.

5. Khan MA, Khan MK. Diagnostic value of HLA-B27 testing in ankylosing spondylitis and Reiter's syndrome. *Ann Intern Med.* 1982;96:70–76.

6. Khan MA. HLA-B27 and its pathogenic role. *J Clin Rheumatol.* 2008;14(1): 50–52.

7. Khan MA. Ankylosing spondylitis: clinical features. In Hochberg M, Silman A, Smolen J, Weinblatt M, Weisman M, eds. *Rheumatology*, 3rd ed. London: Mosby: A Division of Harcourt Health Sciences Ltd.; 2003:1161–1181.

Suggested reading

Feldtkeller E, Khan MA, van der Linden S, van der Heijde D, Braun J. Age at disease onset and diagnosis delay in HLA-B27 negative vs. positive patients with ankylosing spondylitis. *Rheumatol Int.* 2003;23:61–66.

Khan MA. Five classical clinical papers on ankylosing spondylitis. In Dieppe P, Khan MA. HLA-B27 and its subtypes in world populations. *Curr Opin Rheumatol.* 1995;7:263–269.

Khan MA, Ball EJ. Ankylosing spondylitis and genetic aspects. *Best Pract Res Clin Rheumatol.* 2002;16:675–690.

Walsh B, Yocum D, Khan MA. Arthritis and HLA-B27 in North American tribes. *Curr Opin Rheumatol.* 1998;10:319–325.

Wollheim FA, Schumacher HR, eds. *Classical Papers in Rheumatology.* London: Martin Dunitz Ltd.; 2002:118–133.

Chapter 14

Socioeconomic aspects and prognosis

Patients with AS experience reduced vitality and quality of life. Compared with the general population, they are more likely to experience progressive functional impairment over time as well as work disability and possible job loss. Many patients cannot maintain the level of employment that they had before the onset of their disease. Patients with physically demanding jobs are more likely to change their type of work, decrease their work hours, or experience temporary or permanent work disability in contrast to patients who have jobs that are less physically demanding. AS patients leave the labor force at a two- to three-fold higher rate than the general population, and they report similar pain and functional disability as those with RA.[1–4]

All this has a tremendous impact on patients and on society at large in terms of economic costs, both direct and indirect. Moreover, unlike RA, AS usually begins at the prime of one's life, so these patients must deal with the illness for a longer time.[5] Early cessation of employment for patients with AS is associated not only with physically demanding jobs but also with low level of education, complete ossification of the spine, hip joint involvement, acute anterior uveitis, female sex, and the coexistence of nonrheumatic diseases.[1–6]

Economic evaluation of anti-TNF therapy

TNF antagonists are highly effective in AS in alleviating pain and reducing clinical disease activity in both axial and peripheral arthritis, reducing or alleviating extraarticular manifestations, improving quality of life, and maintaining long-term efficacy out to at least 5 years.[2,7–13] The clinical response is greater in patients with earlier stages of disease and less damage.

Recent systematic reviews and economic evaluations of the use of etanercept, infliximab, and adalimumab for the treatment of AS have been published.[8–13] However, we need to obtain robust estimates of the longer-term clinical cost-effectiveness of anti-TNF agents for AS.[8] Incremental cost-effectiveness ratios of adalimumab versus conventional therapy in United Kingdom were estimated to improve with longer time horizons (48 weeks to 5 and 30 years).[14] The central estimate was that over 30 years adalimumab therapy yielded 1.03 more quality-adjusted life-years per patient initiating therapy. This analysis indicates that adalimumab, when used according to U.K. treatment guidelines, is cost-effective compared to conventional therapy for treating AS patients.[14] The short-term (12-month) model showed that the large front-loading of costs makes none of the three biologics appear cost-effective at the currently acceptable threshold, with infliximab yielding much poorer economic results.

Current models make use of costing data obtained from patients with more disabling disease of relatively longer duration and therefore may not reflect the true expected savings of early treatment of patients who otherwise have poor prognoses. We need to identify patients in early stages of their disease, especially those who carry worse prognoses. One might expect that increased awareness of the disease would contribute to shortening of the interval between onset of first symptoms and time of diagnosis, with resultant early treatment with TNF antagonists if treatment with NSAIDs fails. It is expected that earlier intervention in many cases will delay or prevent disability, including loss of working capacity, resulting in considerable savings with regard to the indirect costs due to AS. Unfortunately, many patients who meet the criteria for anti-TNF treatment according to the published guidelines do not receive this treatment for one reason or another (including cost and possible side effects).

A recent review of the clinical effects of these biologicals, based on a review of nine placebo-controlled, randomized, controlled trials (two of adalimumab, five of etanercept, and two of infliximab) found that at 12 weeks, ASAS50 responses were 3.6-fold more likely with TNF blockers than with placebo (along with conventional management).[8] Compared with baseline, BASDAI and BASFI were both reduced by close to 2 points, indicating significant improvement in symptoms and function.

Prognosis

Poor response or intolerance to NSAIDs and the presence of severe extraarticular complications worsen the prognosis. The stage of AS at diagnosis and initiation of appropriate therapy, the severity of early stages of the disease, the quality of medical management, and the degree of patient compliance with the suggested treatment also influence the prognosis. Functional disability progresses more rapidly in older patients and smokers and less rapidly in those who have better social support and who can vperform back exercises regularly. Radiological damage to the cervical and lumbar spine, thoracic wedging, and disease activity are determinants of hyperkyphosis in patients with AS.[15]

An excess mortality was observed in the past, primarily ascribed to amyloidosis and complications of spinal irradiation (excess malignancies, especially a five-fold increase in leukemias). In subsequent studies an excess mortality was observed among nonirradiated patients seen at tertiary care centers, primarily due to cardiopulmonary causes, but only after a period of more than 20 years after their disease diagnosis.[16] These studies involved patients with disease severe enough to impel them to seek specialized care and to be correctly diagnosed at a time when AS was considered a rare disease. Spinal fracture; cardiopulmonary involvement; associated comorbidities, including psoriasis, ulcerative colitis, and Crohn's disease; and complications of medical and surgical treatment all contribute to premature mortality.[1,16,17] It is possible that the survival of patients with mild disease who are diagnosed early and receive appropriate and more effective treatment may be comparable to that of the general population.

References

1. Boonen A, Chorus A, Miedema H, et al. Withdrawal from labour force due to work disability in patients with ankylosing spondylitis. *Ann Rheum Dis*. 2001;60(11):1033–1039.

2. Khan MA. Ankylosing spondylitis: burden of illness, diagnosis, and effective treatment. *J Rheumatol Suppl*. 2006;78:1–33.

3. Ward MM, Reveille JD, Learch TJ, Davis JC Jr, Weisman MH. Impact of ankylosing spondylitis on work and family life: comparisons with the US population. *Arthritis Rheum*. 2008;59(4):497–503.

4. Barlow JH, Wright CC, Williams B, Keat A. Work disability among people with ankylosing spondylitis. *Arthritis Rheum*. 2001;45(5):424–429.

5. Verstappen SM, Jacobs JW, van der Heijde DM, et al. Utility and direct costs: ankylosing spondylitis compared with rheumatoid arthritis. *Ann Rheum Dis*. 2007;66(6):727–731.

6. Ward MM, Kuzis S. Risk factors for work disability in patients with ankylosing spondylitis. *J Rheumatol*. 2001;28(2):315–321.

7. Braun J, Baraliakos X, Listing J, et al. Persistent clinical efficacy and safety of anti-tumour necrosis factor alpha therapy with infliximab in patients with ankylosing spondylitis over 5 years: evidence for different types of response. *Ann Rheum Dis*. 2008;67(3):340–345.

8. McLeod C, Bagust A, Boland A, et al. Adalimumab, etanercept and infliximab for the treatment of ankylosing spondylitis: a systematic review and economic evaluation. *Health Technol Assess*. 2007;11(28):1–158.

9. Kavanaugh A. Economic issues with new rheumatologic therapeutics. *Curr Opin Rheumatol*. 2007;19(3):272–276.

10. Kavanaugh A. The pharmacoeconomics of newer therapeutics for rheumatic diseases. *Rheum Dis Clin North Am*. 2006;32(1):45–56.

11. Han C, Smolen J, Kavanaugh A, et al. The impact of infliximab treatment on quality of life in patients with inflammatory rheumatic diseases. *Arthritis Res Ther*. 2007;9(5):R103.

12. Davis JC, Revicki D, van der Heijde DM, et al. Health-related quality of life outcomes in patients with active AS treated with adalimumab: results from a randomized controlled study. *Arthritis Rheum*. 2007;57(6):1050–1057.

13. Davis JC, van der Heijde D, Dougados M, Woolley JM. Reductions in health-related quality of life in patients with AS and improvements with etanercept therapy. *Arthritis Rheum*. 2005;53(4):494–501.

14. Botteman MF, Hay JW, Luo MP, Curry AS, Wong RL, van Hout BA. Cost effectiveness of adalimumab for the treatment of ankylosing spondylitis in the United Kingdom. *Rheumatology (Oxford)*. 2007;46(8):1320–1328.

15. Vosse D, van der Heijde D, Landewé R, et al. Determinants of hyperkyphosis in patients with ankylosing spondylitis. *Ann Rheum Dis.* 2006;65(6):770–774.

16. Khan MA, Khan MK, Kushner I. Survival among patients with ankylosing spondylitis: a life-table analysis. *J Rheumatol.* 1981;8:86–90.

17. Bakland G, Nossent HC, Gran JT. Incidence and prevalence of ankylosing spondylitis in Northern Norway. *Arthritis Rheum.* 2005;53(6):850–855.

Chapter 15

Brief illustrative case histories

Case 1

A 26-year-old college student was seen with chronic back and hip pain and stiffness for 18 months. The pain was initially felt in the buttocks and hips for the first few months and then progressed to also involve the low back area, and it has been associated with stiffness. His back pain and stiffness are worsened with prolonged sitting and during the second half of the night, as well as on waking up in the morning. The morning stiffness and pain start easing up after 40 minutes, after physical activity or exercise, and after a hot shower. In the past 3 months he has noted pain in the lower rib cage that is accentuated on coughing or sneezing.

He denies any history of chronic diarrhea, skin disease, eye inflammation, or back injury. He is an only child; his father died in a car accident at age 30. A paternal uncle has had a stiff back and neck for many years.

On physical examination, he has tenderness over the sacroiliac joints, lumbar spine, anterior chest wall, and right temporomandibular joint, and limitation of motion of his lumbar spine. His chest expansion on full inspiration is normal, as is the rest of his physical examination. His BASDAI score is 3 on a scale of 0 to 10.

Because of a strong probability of AS based on the clinical findings, a radiograph of the pelvis was ordered. The presence of bilateral sacroiliitis confirmed the diagnosis of AS.

An NSAID was prescribed to be taken twice a day with food. He was encouraged to stay active, to swim regularly, and to follow a regular exercise regimen. His illness was explained and he was given counseling. He was also given a pamphlet about AS and online information about self-help groups and organizations for AS patients because he is computer literate. His symptoms were much better when he was seen 2 weeks later, and his BASDAI score had decreased to 2.5.

In patients with AS, assessment of pain, physical function, spinal mobility (including chest expansion); duration of morning stiffness; presence of inflamed peripheral joints; and enthesitis are critical elements to follow over time. Laboratory tests, such as CRP and ESR, and musculoskeletal imaging can also help in assessing and monitoring disease activity and severity.

In 1990, at age 18, this patient began complaining about chronic hip and low back pain of insidious onset, without any history of physical injury to his back. In 1993 he visited a chiropractor, but his symptoms worsened after spinal manipulation. In 1994 he saw his primary care physician, who prescribed ibuprofen, but it did not help. His medication was changed to naproxen (Naprosyn) 500 mg bid, but he developed a peptic ulcer that required hospitalization and treatment with cimetidine (Tagamet). He was advised not to take Naprosyn or other NSAIDs. A spinal radiograph was read as normal.

In 1997 he changed doctors and was treated with 5-day course of methylprednisone; it did not help. He was started on oxycodone with acetaminophen (Percocet) and later prednisone 20 mg daily, but his symptoms persisted.

In 1998 he was referred to an orthopedist for his complaints of low back pain with radiation down the upper part of both legs but not below his knees. Spinal radiographs were repeated and he was diagnosed with a herniated disc. He underwent back surgery, but it did not help.

In 2000 he was prescribed celecoxib (Celebrex) 200 mg twice daily with food and was advised to swim regularly; it helped his back pain to some extent. Later that year, in addition to his chronic back pain and stiffness, he also started having neck pain and stiffness.

In 2001 the patient was referred to a rheumatologist, who noted flattening of the lumbar spine with limitation of lumbar and cervical spine motion and decreased chest expansion. There was no tenderness of the sacroiliac joints or spine. He had no psoriasis but did have occasional loose bowel movements. His family history was noncontributory. His ESR was 25, CRP was 1.3, and a pelvic radiograph showed a fused right sacroiliac joint; his left sacroiliac joint was only partially fused. He was diagnosed with AS and was prescribed methotrexate and folic acid. The dosage of methotrexate was gradually increased to 17.5 mg once weekly, but the patient did not notice any benefit.

In 2002 the patient complained of worsening neck pain. His HLA-B27 test was negative, and his gastrointestinal workup was negative for Crohn's disease or ulcerative colitis. He was prescribed narcotics for pain relief, and prednisone 10 mg daily was added, but it did not provide any benefit. Sulfasalazine was then added, but he could not tolerate it because of its gastrointestinal effects.

In 2003 the patient consulted another rheumatologist who noted that his BASDAI score was 7.4 and, after a thorough evaluation and patient education about therapeutic options, started him on a TNF antagonist. Improvement was marked, and after 12 weeks the BASDAI score had dropped to 3.4. He was weaned off his other medications except celecoxib.

In 2005, because of a change of job and subsequent change in his health insurance, the new insurance company denied the patient continuation of his previous TNF antagonist therapy, which resulted in worsening of his symptoms. The patient was started on a different TNF antagonist; it controlled his spinal pain and stiffness within 4 weeks.

Case 3

A 41-year-old white woman presented with chronic low back pain and stiffness that had worsened during the preceding 2 years. Her back pain and stiffness become worse after inactivity and wake her up late at night and early in the morning. She feels better after physical activity and exercise. She also has had chest pain that is accentuated by sneezing and coughing. Her back has gradually been becoming stiffer over the past 2 years, which has caused her difficulty in performing activities of daily living.

The onset of low back pain was preceded by episodic upper back pain (between the shoulder blades) and sometimes neck pain for 10 years, for which she had seen many doctors and had many tests, including radiographs and bone scans. She had been previously treated with full doses of different NSAIDs without much relief from her symptoms. She was told that she had fibromyalgia.

Her personal and family medical histories were unremarkable. She had been seeing her ophthalmologist because of occasional recurrent episodes of HLA-B27-associated acute anterior uveitis (acute iritis) during the past 20 years.

On examination she walked with a slightly stiff gait. She had tenderness over the lower cervical spinal processes, over the whole thoracolumbar spine, and over both sacroiliac joints. She had diminished lumbar spinal motion in all planes (Schober's test showed only 2 cm of mobility). Her neck motion was decreased in all planes. Chest expansion was only 3 cm. Her BASDAI score was 6, indicating active disease.

Laboratory tests showed elevations of ESR and CRP. A recent radiograph of the pelvis did not show definite evidence of sacroiliitis. An MRI (STIR technique and without gadolinium enhancement) clearly showed areas of edema of the sacrum and ilium adjacent to both sacroiliac joints, indicative of bilateral sacroiliitis and confirming the clinical diagnosis of AS. She was treated with a TNF antagonist, with excellent response, and her BASDAI score dropped to 1.4. Her ESR and CRP values normalized.

This case exemplifies the difficulty in establishing a definite diagnosis in the absence of sacroiliitis on a conventional radiograph. It also shows the role of MRI in making the diagnosis of axial undifferentiated spondyloarthropathy ("pre-radiographic AS"). She has had no further episode of acute iritis.

Case 4

A 41-year-old woman from a foreign country presented with severe back pain and stiffness that did not respond to full doses of different NSAIDs.

She had seen many physicians in more than one country, and her pain was thought to be due to active inflammation from her long-standing AS. She stated that she was treated with methotrexate at one stage, which caused hair loss but did not relieve her symptoms. She was told that conventional radiography showed typical changes of advanced AS with bamboo spine.

A review of her clinical history revealed that her back pain was no more inflammatory in type, and it worsened with physical activity and was relieved with inactivity. Physical examination and a review of the radiographs she had brought with her suggested the presence of discitis or pseudarthrosis in her lumbar spine, along with typical changes of advanced AS. Further imaging studies (CT and MRI) showed pseudarthrosis of the mid-lumbar spine, which was the cause of her pain. Initial treatment with a lumbar brace did not provide much relief. She underwent surgery for spinal fusion, which relieved all her pain.

This case exemplifies the importance of being vigilant for the complications of spinal fracture and pseudarthrosis in patients with advanced AS.

Appendix 1

Organizations for AS and related SpA

For physicians

SPARTAN (Spondyloarthritis Research and Treatment Network)

www.spartangroup.org

SPARTAN was founded in 2003 by a group of North American clinicians and researchers to promote research, education, and treatment of AS and related SpA. SPARTAN has held its latest (fifth and sixth) annual research meetings in Cleveland, Ohio, along with an educational pre-meeting conference designed for postgraduate rheumatology fellows in training.[1]

SPARCC (Spondyloarthritis Research Consortium of Canada)

SPARCC is a Canadaian consortium with aims very similar to those of SPARTAN.

ASAS (Assessment of Spondyloarthritis International Society)

www.asas-group.org

ASAS is an international society of experts in the field of SpA. Its mission is to support and promote translational and clinical research of SpA, with the goal of improving the well-being and outcome of patients with SpA. The means to achieve this goal include the following:

- Increasing awareness of SpA
- Facilitating early diagnosis
- Developing and validating assessment tools
- Evaluating treatment modalities

GRAPPA (Group for Research and Assessment of Psoriasis and Psoriatic Arthritis)

www.grappanetwork.org

For patients

ASIF (Ankylosing Spondylitis International Federation)

www.asif.rheumanet.org and www.spondylitis-international.org

ASIF is a worldwide organization of national self-help societies of patients with AS and related SpA, established in 1988 to increase public awareness and knowledge of these diseases around the world. Its aims are as follows:

- Exchange of information and experiences among the member societies
- Cooperation in international research projects
- Exchange of articles for publication in the journals of the member societies
- Support of newly formed societies
- Establishment of contacts with spondylitis patients in countries where an AS society does not yet exist

Questionnaires such as BASDAI, BASFI, and BASMI can be downloaded as PDF files from ASIF's Web site (www.spondylitis-international.org); they can be found under "Practical forms for the assessment of AS." ASIF has also published illustrated booklets; one of them describes assessment scores and disease criteria, and another addresses the special considerations relating to automobile driving for patients with AS.

ASIF maintains at its Web site an up-to-date list of the many patient support groups and organizations in various countries. The **Spondylitis Association of America (SAA)** maintains a Web site (www.spondylitis.org) that is very informative and frequently updated. **The National AS Society (NASS)** of the United Kingdom also has a Web site (www.nass.co.uk).

The aims of these national patient support groups and organizations are as follows:

- Improve the physical and mental health of patients with AS or related diseases and organize supervised exercise and recreational therapy groups
- Allow patients to discuss their experiences and prevent social isolation
- Advise patients about social, medical, and work-related problems associated with their disease
- Cooperate with physicians and allied health professionals and promote and encourage research into the diseases
- Represent the interests of the patients in legal and health-care arenas
- Increase public awareness about the diseases in their countries

ASIM (Ankylosing Spondylitis International Matrix)
www.hlab27.com

Reference

1. Colbert RA, Deodhar AA, Khan MA, et al. 2007 Annual Research and Education Meeting of the Spondyloarthritis Research and Therapy Network (SPARTAN). *J Rheumatol.* 2008;35(7):1398–1402.

Appendix 2

Author's selected publications in the field of AS and related SpA

Books and book chapters

- Akkoc N, Khan MA. Epidemiology of ankylosing spondylitis and related spondyloarthropathies. In Weisman MH, Reveille JD, van der Heijde D, eds. *Ankylosing Spondylitis and the Spondyloarthropathies: A Companion to Rheumatology.* London: Mosby-Elsevier; 2006:117–131.
- Braun J, Sieper J, Khan MA. Recent advances in pharmacotherapy of spondyloarthropathies. In Tsokos GC, Kammer GM, Moreland LW, Pelletier J, Gay S, eds. *Modern Therapeutics in Rheumatic Diseases.* Totowa, NJ: Humana Press; 2002:595–603.
- Dougados M, Revel M, Khan MA. Management of spondyloarthropathy. In van de Putte LBA, Williams HJ, van Riel P, Furst DE, eds. *Therapy of Systemic Rheumatic Disorders.* New York: Marcel Dekker; 1998:375–406.
- Elyan M, Khan MA. Spondyloarthropathies. In *Clinical Care in the Rheumatic Diseases,* 3rd ed. Atlanta: Association of Rheumatology Health Professionals; 2006:177–185.
- Elyan M, Khan MA. Spondyloarthropathies. In *Spinal Cord Medicine Textbook: Musculoskeletal Care,* 2008 (in press).
- Khan MA. Ankylosing spondylitis. In Calin A, ed. *Spondyloarthropathies.* New York: Grune & Stratton; 1984:69–117.
- Khan MA. Spondyloarthropathies in non-Caucasians. In Calin A, ed. *Spondyloarthropathies.* New York: Grune & Stratton; 1984:265–277.
- Khan MA. How the B27 test can help in the diagnosis of spondyloarthropathies. In Calin A, ed. *Spondyloarthropathies.* New York: Grune & Stratton; 1984:323–337.
- Khan MA. Spondyloarthropathies in non-Caucasian populations of the world. In Ziff M, Cohen SB, eds. *The Spondyloarthropathies* (Advances in Inflammation Research, vol. 9). New York: Raven Press; 1985:91–99.
- Khan MA. HLA and ankylosing spondylitis. In Calabro JJ, Dick C, eds. *Ankylosing Spondylitis: New Clinical Applications in Rheumatology,* vol. 1. Lancaster, UK: MTP Press Limited; 1987:23–44.

- Khan MA. Heterogeneity and a wider spectrum of ankylosing spondylitis and related disorders. In Lipsky PE, Taurog JD, eds. *HLA-B27+ Spondyloarthropathies*. New York: Elsevier; 1991:133–143.

- Khan MA. Ankylosing spondylitis. In Schumacher HR Jr, ed. *Primer on the Rheumatic Diseases*, 10th ed. Atlanta: Arthritis Foundation; 1993:154–158.

- Khan MA. Ankylosing spondylitis: clinical features. In Klippel JH, Dieppe PA, eds. *Rheumatology*. London: Mosby-Year Book Europe Ltd.; 1994:3.25.1–3.25.10.

- Khan MA. Ankylosing spondylitis. In Rakel RE, ed. *Conn's Current Therapy*. Philadelphia: WB Saunders; 1994:957–959.

- Khan MA. Ankylosing spondylitis: clinical features. In Klippel JH, Dieppe PA, eds. *Rheumatology*. London: Mosby-Year Book Europe Ltd.; 1995:211–220.

- Khan MA. Prevalence of HLA-B27 in world populations. In Lopez-Larrea C, ed. *HLA-B27 in the Development of Spondyloarthropathies*. Austin, TX: RG Landes; 1997:95–112.

- Khan MA. Spondyloarthropathies. In *Rheumatology MKSAP (Medical Knowledge Self-Assessment Program)*, 2nd ed. Developed by the American College of Rheumatology and the American College of Physicians, 1997:126–139.

- Khan MA. Axial pain syndromes: back and neck pain. In *Rheumatology MKSAP (Medical Knowledge Self-Assessment Program)*, 2nd ed. Developed by the American College of Rheumatology and the American College of Physicians, 1997:258–266.

- Khan MA. Ankylosing spondylitis. In *Primer on the Rheumatic Diseases*, 11th ed. Atlanta: Arthritis Foundation; 1997:189–193.

- Khan MA. Ankylosing spondylitis: clinical features. In Klippel JH, Dieppe PA, eds. *Rheumatology*, 2nd ed. London: Mosby-Wolfe; 1998:6.16.1– 6.16.10.

- Khan MA. Seronegative spondyloarthropathies. In Home HS, Feng PH, eds. *Textbook of Clinical Rheumatology*. Singapore: National Arthritis Foundation; 1998:125–147.

- Khan MA. Ankylosing spondylitis—the clinical aspects. In Calin A, Taurog J, eds. *The Spondylarthritides*. Oxford: Oxford University Press; 1998:27–40.

- Khan MA. A worldwide overview—the epidemiology of HLA-B27 and associated spondyloarthritides. In Calin A, Taurog J, eds. *The Spondylarthritides*. Oxford: Oxford University Press; 1998:17–26.

- Khan MA. Spondyloarthropathies. In Hunder G, ed. *Atlas of Rheumatology*. Philadelphia: Current Science; 1998:5.1–5.24.

- Khan MA. Back and neck pain. In Fitzgerald F, ed. *Current Practice of Medicine*, 2nd ed. Philadelphia: Current Medicine; 1999:187–203.

- Khan MA. Ankylosing spondylitis. In Rakel RE, ed. *Conn's Current Therapy*. Philadelphia: WB Saunders; 1999:994–996.

- Khan MA. Five classical clinical papers on ankylosing spondylitis. In Dieppe P, Wollheim FA, Schumacher HR, eds. *Classical Papers in Rheumatology*. London: Martin Dunitz Ltd.; 2002:118–133.

- Khan MA. *Ankylosing Spondylitis: The Facts*. Oxford: Oxford University Press; 2002.
- Khan MA. HLA-B27 und seine Subtypen. In Braun J, Sieper J, eds. *Spondylitis Ankylosans*. Bremen: Unimed Verlag AG; 2002:64–69.
- Khan MA. Spondyloarthropathies. In Hunder G, ed. *Atlas of Rheumatology*, 3rd ed. Philadelphia: Current Medicine; 2002:141–167.
- Khan MA. Ankylosing spondylitis: clinical features. In Hochberg M, Silman A, Smolen J, Weinblatt M, Weisman M, eds. *Rheumatology*, 3rd ed. London: Mosby: A Division of Harcourt Health Sciences Ltd.; 2003:1161–1181.
- Khan MA. Spondyloarthropathies. In Hunder G, ed. *Atlas of Rheumatology*, 4th ed. Philadelphia: Current Medicine; 2005:151–180.
- Khan MA. Patient's perspective. In van Royen BJ, Dijkmans BAC, eds. *Ankylosing Spondylitis: Diagnosis and Management*. New York: Taylor & Francis; 2006:95–97.
- Khan MA, Kammer G. Laboratory findings and pathology of psoriatic arthritis. In Gerber LH, Espinoza L, eds. *Psoriatic Arthritis*. New York: Grune & Stratton; 1985:109–124.
- Khan MA, Kushner I. Diagnosis of ankylosing spondylitis. In Cohen AS, ed. *Progress in Clinical Rheumatology*, vol. 1. New York: Grune & Stratton; 1984:145–178.
- Khan MA, McGonagle D. State of the art review: pathogenesis of anky-losing spondylitis and related spondyloarthropathies. In Emery P, ed. *Fast Facts in Rheumatology*. Oxford: Health Press; 1999:61–66.
- Khan MA, Sieper J. Reactive arthritis. In Koopman WJ, Moreland LW, eds. *Arthritis and Allied Conditions*, 15th ed. Philadelphia: Lippincott Williams & Wilkins; 2004:1335–1355.
- Khan MA, Skosey JL. Ankylosing spondylitis and related spondyloarthrop-athies. In Samter M, Talmage DW, Frank MM, Austen KF, Claman HN, eds. *Immunological Diseases*, 4th ed. Boston: Little, Brown & Company; 1988:1509–1538.
- Khan MA, Wilber RG. Back and neck pain. In Bone R, ed. *Current Practice of Medicine*. Philadelphia: Current Medicine; 1996:VI:8.1–VI:8.14.
- van der Linden SM, Khan MA. Spondyloarthropathies. In Wigley RD, ed. *The Primary Prevention of Rheumatic Diseases*. New York: Parthenon Publishing Group; 1993:221–228.

Other selected relevant publications

- Amor B, Dougados M, Khan MA. Management of refractory ankylosing spondylitis and related spondylarthropathies. *Rheum Dis Clin North Am*. 1995;21:117–128.
- Ahmed Q, Chung-Park M, Mustafa K, Khan MA. Psoriatic spondyloar-thropathy with secondary amyloidosis. *J Rheumatol*. 1996;23:1107–1110.
- Akkoc N, Khan MA. Etiopathogenic role of HLA-B27 alleles in ankylosing spondylitis. *APLAR J Rheumatol*. 2005;8:146–153.

- Akkoc N, van der Linden S, Khan MA. Ankylosing spondylitis and symptom-modifying vs. disease-modifying therapy. *Best Pract Res Clin Rheumatol*. 2006;20(3):539–557.
- Ball EJ, Khan MA. HLA-B27 polymorphism. *Bone Joint Spine*. 2001;68:378–382.
- Braun J, Khan MA, Sieper J. Entheses and enthesopathy: what is the target of the immune response? *Ann Rheum Dis*. 2000;59:985–994.
- Braun J, van der Heijde D, Dougados M, et al. Staging of patients with ankylosing spondylitis: a preliminary proposal. *Ann Rheum Dis*. 2002;61(Suppl 3): iii19–iii23.
- Cats A, van der Linden SM, Goei The HS, Khan MA. Proposals for diagnostic criteria of ankylosing spondylitis and allied disorders. *Clin Exp Rheumatol*. 1987;5:167–171.
- Colbert RA, Deodhar AA, Khan MA, et al. 2007 Annual Research and Education Meeting of the Spondyloarthritis Research and Therapy Network (SPARTAN). *J Rheumatol*. 2008;35(7):1398–1402.
- Dejelo CL, Braun WE, Khan MA, Clough JD. HLA-DR antigens and ankylosing spondylitis. *Transplant Proc*. 1978;10:971–972.
- Dougados M, Dijkmanns B, Khan MA, Maksymowych W, van der Linden S. Conventional treatments for ankylosing spondylitis. *Ann Rheum Dis*. 2002;61 (Suppl 3):iii40–iii50.
- Dougados M, Revel M, Khan MA. Spondylarthropathy treatment: progress in medical treatment, physical therapy and rehabilitation. *Ballieres Clin Rheumatol*. 1998;12:717–736.
- Elyan M, Khan MA. The role of non-steroidal anti-inflammatory medications and exercise in the treatment of ankylosing spondylitis. *Curr Rheumatol Rep*. 2006;8:255–259.
- Elyan M, Khan MA. Diagnosing ankylosing spondylitis. *J Rheumatol*. 2006;33(Suppl 78):12–23.
- Elyan M, Khan MA. Is low-dose infliximab every 8 weeks effective in treating ankylosing spondylitis? *Curr Rheumatol Rep*. 2007;9(5):351–352.
- Elyan M, Khan MA. Another look at low-dose infliximab in treating ankylosing spondylitis. *Curr Rheumatol Rep*. 2007;9(5):352.
- Elyan M, Khan MA. Sulfasalazine in undifferentiated spondyloarthropathies. *Curr Rheumatol Rep*. 2007;9(5):349–350.
- Elyan M, Khan MA. Does physical therapy have a place in the treatment of ankylosing spondylitis? *Curr Opin Rheumatol*. 2008;20(3):282–286.
- Feldtkeller E, Bruckel J, Khan MA. Scientific contributions of the ankylosing spondylitis patient advocacy groups. *Curr Opin Rheumatol*. 2000;12:239–247.
- Feldtkeller E, Khan MA, van der Linden S, van der Heijde D, Braun J. Age at disease onset and diagnosis delay in HLA-B27-negative vs. -positive patients with ankylosing spondylitis. *Rheumatol Int*. 2003;23:61–66.

- Feltkamp TE, Khan MA, Lopez de Castro JA. The pathogenic role of HLA-B27. *Immunology Today.* 1996;17:5–7.
- François RJ, Braun J, Khan MA. Entheses and enthesitis: a histopathological review and relevance to spondyloarthropathies. *Curr Opin Rheumatol.* 2001;13:255–264.
- Gladman DD, Inman RD, Cook RR, et al. International Spondyloarthritis Inter-Observer Reliability Exercise—The INSPIRE Study: I. Assessment of Spinal Measures. *J Rheumatol.* 2007;34(8):1733–1739.
- Gladman DD, Inman RD, Cook RR, et al. International Spondyloarthritis Inter-Observer Reliability Exercise—The INSPIRE Study: II. Assessment of peripheral joints, enthesitis and dactylitis. *J Rheumatol.* 2007;34(8):1740–1745.
- Granfors K, Märker-Hermann E, De Keyser P, Khan MA, Veys EM, Yu DT. The cutting edge of spondyloarthropathy research in the millennium. *Arthritis Rheum.* 2002;46:606–613.
- Hammoudeh M, Khan MA. Genetics of HLA associated diseases: ankylosing spondylitis. *J Rheumatol.* 1983;10:301–304.
- Jin L, Weisman M, Zhang G, et al. Lack of linkage of IL1RN genotype with ankylosing spondylitis susceptibility. *Arthritis Rheum.* 2004;50:3047–3048.
- Jin L, Weisman M, Zhang G, et al. Lack of association of MMP3 with ankylosing spondylitis susceptibility. *Rheumatology.* 2005;44:55–60.
- Jumshyd A, Khan MA. Ankylosing hyperostosis in American Blacks: a longitudinal study. *Clin Rheumatol.* 1983;2:123–126.
- Khan MA. Race-related differences in HLA association with ankylosing spondylitis and Reiter's disease in American Blacks and Whites. *J Natl Med Assoc.* 1978;70:41–42.
- Khan MA. Clinical application of HLA-B27 test in rheumatic diseases: a current perspective. *Arch Intern Med.* 1980;140:177–180.
- Khan MA. Axial arthropathy in Whipple's disease. *J Rheumatol.* 1982;9:928–929.
- Khan MA. B7-CREG and ankylosing spondylitis. *Br J Rheumatol.* 1983;22(Supp 2):129–132.
- Khan MA. A double-blind comparison of diclofenac and indomethacin in the treatment of ankylosing spondylitis. *J Rheumatol.* 1987;14:118–123.
- Khan MA. Immunogenetics of ankylosing spondylitis: clinically oriented aspects. *Clin Exp Rheumatol.* 1987;5(Suppl 1):S49–S52.
- Khan MA. Genetics of HLA-B27. *Br J Rheumatol.* 1988;27(Suppl II):6–11.
- Khan MA. Ankylosing spondylitis and heterogeneity of HLA-B27. *Semin Arthritis Rheum.* 1988;18:134–141.
- Khan MA. Editorial comment: HLA-B27 testing in ankylosing spondylitis: an analysis of the pretesting assumptions. *J Rheumatol.* 1989;16:634–636.
- Khan MA. Newer clinical and radiographic manifestations of the seronegative spondyloarthropathies. *Curr Opin Rheumatol.* 1989;1:139–143.
- Khan MA. An overview of the HLA system. *Spine: State of the Art Reviews.* 1990;4:595–605.

- Khan MA. Medical and surgical treatment of spondyloarthropathies. *Curr Opin Rheumatol.* 1990;2:592–599.
- Khan MA. An overview of clinical spectrum and heterogeneity of spondyloarthropathies. *Rheum Dis Clin North Am.* 1992;18:1–10.
- Khan MA. Etiopathogenesis of ankylosing spondylitis. *Rheumatol Rev.* 1993;2:67–71.
- Khan MA. Spondyloarthropathies: editorial overview. *Curr Opin Rheumatol.* 1993;5:405–407.
- Khan MA. Pathogenesis of ankylosing spondylitis: recent advances [editorial]. *J Rheumatol.* 1993;20:1273–1277.
- Khan MA. Spondyloarthropathies: editorial overview. *Curr Opin Rheumatol.* 1994;6:351–353.
- Khan MA. HLA-B27 and its subtypes in world populations. *Curr Opin Rheumatol.* 1995;7:263–269.
- Khan MA. Arthritis and autoimmunity: report on the 15th Sigrid Juselius Symposium. *Rheumatol Int.* 1995;15:39–42.
- Khan MA. Epidemiology of HLA-B27 and arthritis. *Clin Rheumatol.* 1996;15(Suppl 1):10–12.
- Khan MA. Editorial review: spondyloarthropathies/spondyloarthritides. *Curr Opin Rheumatol.* 1996;8:267–268.
- Khan MA. Spondyloarthropathies: editorial review. *Curr Opin Rheumatol.* 1997;9:281–283.
- Khan MA. Slow-acting anti-rheumatic drugs in severe ankylosing spondylitis [editorial]. *J Clin Rheumatol.* 1998;4:109–111.
- Khan MA. Spondyloarthropathies: editorial overview. *Curr Opin Rheumatol.* 1998;10:279–281.
- Khan MA. Spondyloarthropathies: editorial overview. *Curr Opin Rheumatol.* 1999;11:233–234.
- Khan MA. HLA-B27 polymorphism and association with disease [editorial]. *J Rheumatol.* 2000;27:1110–1114.
- Khan MA. Patient-doctor. *Ann Intern Med.* 2000;133:233–235.
- Khan MA. Update: the twenty subtypes of HLA-B27. *Curr Opin Rheumatol.* 2000;12:239–247.
- Khan MA. My self-portrait. *Clin Rheumatol.* 2001;20:1–2.
- Khan MA. Update on spondyloarthropathies. *Ann Intern Med.* 2002;136:896–907.
- Khan MA. Introductory comments. New treatment strategies in ankylosing spondylitis. *Ann Rheum Dis.* 2002;61(Suppl 3):iii3–iii7.
- Khan MA. Ankylosing spondylitis—the history of medical therapies. *Clin Exp Rheumatol.* 2002;20(Suppl 28):S3–S5.
- Khan MA. Thoughts concerning the early diagnosis of ankylosing spondylitis and related diseases. *Clin Exp Rheumatol.* 2002;20(Suppl 28):S6–S10.
- Khan MA. The perspective of two paintings by a patient-physician. *J Medicine and the Person.* 2005;3(2):83–84.

- Khan MA (ed.). Ankylosing spondylitis: burden of illness, diagnosis, and effective treatment. *J Rheumatol* . 2006;33(Suppl 78):1–31.

- Khan MA. Ankylosing spondylitis: a dual perspective of the current issues and challenges. *J Rheumatol*. 2006;33(Suppl 78):1–3.

- Khan MA. HLA-B27 and its pathogenic role. *J Clin Rheumatol*. 2008;14(1):50–52.

- Khan MA, Akkoc N. Commentary: ten key recommendations for the management of ankylosing spondylitis. *Nature Clin Pract Rheumatol*. 2006;2(9):468–469.

- Khan MA, Askari AD, Braun WE, Aponte CJ. Low association of HLA-B27 with Reiter's syndrome in Blacks. *Ann Intern Med*. 1979;90:202–203.

- Khan MA, Ball EJ. Ankylosing spondylitis and genetic aspects. *Best Pract Res Clin Rheumatol*. 2002;16:675–690.

- Khan MA, Braun WE, Kushner I, Grecek DE, Muir WA, Steinberg AG. HLA-B27 in ankylosing spondylitis: differences in frequency and relative risk in American Blacks and Caucasians. *J Rheumatol*. 1977;4(Suppl 3): 39–43.

- Khan MA, Clegg DO, Deodhar AA, et al. Meeting report. 2006 Annual Research and Education Meeting of the Spondyloarthritis Research and Therapy Network (SPARTAN). *J Rheumatol*. 2007;34(5):1118–1124.

- Khan MA, Kellner H. Immunogenetics of spondyloarthropathies. *Rheum Dis Clin North Am*. 1992;18:837–864.

- Khan MA, Khan MK. Diagnostic value of HLA-B27 testing in ankylosing spondylitis and Reiter's syndrome. *Ann Intern Med*. 1982;96:70–76.

- Khan MA, Khan MK. HLA-B27 as an aid to diagnosis of ankylosing spondylitis. *Spine: State of the Art Reviews*. 1990;4:617–625.

- Khan MA, Khan MK, Kushner I. Survival among patients with ankylosing spondylitis: a life-table analysis. *J Rheumatol*. 1981;8:86–90.

- Khan MA, Kushner I. Ankylosing spondylitis and multiple sclerosis: a possible association. *Arthritis Rheum*. 1979;22:784–786.

- Khan MA, Kushner I, Braun WE. Comparison of clinical features of HLA-B27 positive and negative patients with ankylosing spondylitis. *Arthritis Rheum*. 1977;20:909–912.

- Khan MA, Kushner I, Braun WE. Genetic heterogeneity in primary ankylosing spondylitis. *J Rheumatol*. 1980;7:383–386.

- Khan MA, Kushner I, Braun WE, Zachary AA, Steinberg AG. HLA-B27 homozygosity in ankylosing spondylitis: relationship to risk and severity. *Tissue Antigens*. 1978;11:434–438.

- Khan MA, Kushner I, Freehafer AA. Sacroiliac joint abnormalities in paraplegics. *Ann Rheum Dis*. 1979;38:317–319.

- Khan MA, Lai J-H, Chou C-T, Chang D-M, Liu H-C. Spinal fractures in ankylosing spondylitis. *J Musculoskeletal Med*. 1993;10:45–57.

- Khan MA, Mathieu A, Sorrentino R, Akkoc N. The pathogenic role of HLA-B27 and its subtypes in ankylosing spondylitis. *Autoimmunity Rev*. 2007;6(3):183–189.

- Khan MA, van der Linden SM. A wider spectrum of spondyloarthropathies. *Semin Arthritis Rheum.* 1990;20:107–113.
- Khan MA, van der Linden SM. Ankylosing spondylitis and associated diseases. *Rheum Dis Clin North Am.* 1990;16:551–579.
- Khan MA, van der Linden SM. Ankylosing spondylitis: clinical aspects. *Spine: State of the Art Reviews.* 1990;4:529–551.
- Khan, MA, van der Linden SM. Undifferentiated spondyloarthropathies. *Spine: State of the Art Reviews.* 1990;4:657–664.
- Khan MA, van der Linden SM, Kushner I, Valkenburg HA, Cats A. Spondylitic disease without radiological evidence of sacroiliitis in relatives of HLA-B27 positive patients. *Arthritis Rheum.* 1985;28:40–43.
- Khan MA, Wolfe F, Kleinheksel SM, Molta C. HLA DR4 and B27 antigens in familial and sporadic rheumatoid arthritis. *Scand J Rheumatol.* 1987;16:433–436.
- Kahn M-F, Khan MA. SAPHO syndrome. *Ballieres Clin Rheumatol.* 1994;8:333–362.
- Mackiewicz A, Khan MA, Gorny A, Kapcinska M, Calabrese LH, Espinoza LR. Glycoforms of α_1-acid glycoprotein in sera of human immunodeficiency virus infected individuals. *J Infect Dis.* 1994;169:1360–1363.
- Mackiewicz A, Khan MA, Reynolds TL, van der Linden S, Kushner I. Serum IgA and acute phase proteins in ankylosing spondylitis. *Ann Rheum Dis.* 1989;48:99–103.
- Martin TM, Zhang G, Luo J, et al. A locus on chromosome 9p predisposes to a specific disease manifestation, acute anterior uveitis, in ankylosing spondylitis, a genetically complex, multisystem, inflammatory disease. *Arthritis Rheum.* 2005;52:269–274.
- McGonagle D, Khan MA, Marzo-Ortega H, O'Connor P, Gibbon W, Emery P. Enthesitis in ankylosing spondylitis and related spondyloarthropathies. *Curr Opin Rheumatol.* 1999;11:244–250.
- Mehra NK, Khan MA, Vaidya MC, Malaviya AN, Batta RK. HLA antigens in acute anterior uveitis and spondyloarthropathies in Asian Indians and their comparison with American Whites and Blacks. *J Rheumatol.* 1983;10:981–984.
- Mijiyawa M, Oniankitan O, Khan MA. Spondyloarthropathies in sub-Saharan Africa. *Curr Opin Rheumatol.* 2000;12:263–268.
- Miron SD, Khan MA, Wiesen E, Kushner I, Bellon EM. The value of quantitative sacroiliac scintigraphy in detection of sacroiliitis. *Clin Rheumatol.* 1983;2:407–414.
- Olafsson S, Khan MA. Musculoskeletal features of acne, hidradenitis suppurativa and dissecting cellulitis of the scalp. *Rheum Dis Clin North Am.* 1992;18:215–224.
- Olivieri I, D'Angelo S, Cutro MS, et al. Diffuse idiopathic skeletal hyperostosis may give the typical postural abnormalities of advanced ankylosing spondylitis. *Rheumatology (Oxford).* 2007;46(11):1709–1711.

- Onen F, Akar S, Birlik M, et al. Prevalence of ankylosing spondylitis and related spondyloarthritis in an urban area of Izmir, Turkey. *J Rheumatol.* 2008;35(2):305–309.

- Payami H, Khan MA, Grennan DM, Sanders PA, Dyer PA, Thomson G. Analysis of genetic interrelationship among HLA-associated diseases. *Am J Hum Genet.* 1987;41:331–349.

- Pazirandeh M, Ziran BH, Khandelwal BK, Reynolds TL, Khan MA. Relapsing polychondritis and spondyloarthropathies. *J Rheumatol.* 1988;15:630–632.

- Pham T, van der Heijde D, Calin A, et al. Initiation of biologics in anky-losing spondylitis patients: results of a Delphi technique within the ASAS group. *Ann Rheum Dis.* 2003;62:812–816.

- Reveille JD, Ball EJ, Khan MA. HLA-B27 and genetic predisposing factors in spondyloarthropathies. *Curr Opin Rheumatol.* 2001;13:265–272.

- Reynolds TL, Khan MA, van der Linden S, Cleveland RP. Differences in HLA-B27-positive and -negative patients with ankylosing spondylitis: study of clinical disease activity and levels of serum IgA, C-reactive pro-tein, and haptoglobin. *Ann Rheum Dis.* 1991;50:154–157.

- Robinson WP, van der Linden SM, Khan MA, et al. HLA-Bw60 increases susceptibility to ankylosing spondylitis in HLA-B27-positive individuals. *Arthritis Rheum.* 1989;32:1135–1141.

- Rudwaleit M, Khan MA, Sieper J. The challenge of diagnosis and classifi-cation in early ankylosing spondylitis: do we need new criteria? *Arthritis Rheum.* 2005;52:1000–1008.

- Rudwaleit M, van der Heijde D, Khan MA, Braun J, Sieper J. How to diag-nose axial spondyloarthropathy early. *Ann Rheum Dis.* 2004;63:535–543.

- Sieper J, Rudwaleit M, Khan MA, Braun J. Concepts and epidemiology of spondyloarthritis. *Best Pract Res Clin Rheumatol.* 2006;20(3):401–417.

- Sun JP, Khan MA, Farhat AZ, Bahler RC. Alterations in cardiac dia-stolic function in patients with ankylosing spondylitis. *Intl J Cardiol.* 1992;37:65–72.

- Thompson GH, Khan MA, Bilenker RM. Spontaneous atlantoaxial sub-luxation as a presenting manifestation of juvenile ankylosing spondylitis. *Spine.* 1982;7:78–79.

- Toivanen A, Khan MA. Therapeutic dilemmas in ankylosing spondylitis and related spondyloarthropathies. *Rheumatol Rev.* 1994;3:21–27.

- van der Heijde D, Bellamy N, Calin A, Dougados M, Khan MA, van der Linden S. Preliminary core sets for endpoints in ankylosing spondylitis. *J Rheumatol.* 1997;24:2225–2229.

- van der Heijde DMFM, Calin A, Dougados M, Khan MA, van der Linden SM, Bellamy N, on behalf of the ASAS working group. Selection of spe-cific instruments for each domain in core set for DC-ART, SM-ARD, physical therapy, and clinical record keeping in ankylosing spondylitis: progress report of ASAS working group. *J Rheumatol.* 1999;26:951–954.

- van der Heijde DMFM, van der Linden SM, Bellamy N, Calin A, Dougados M, Khan MA. Which domains should be included in a core set for endpoints in ankylosing spondylitis? Introduction to the ankylosing spondylitis module of OMERACT IV. *J Rheumatol.* 1999;26:945–947.

- van der Linden S, Cats A, Valkenburg HA, Khan MA. Evaluation of the diagnostic criteria for ankylosing spondylitis: a proposal for modification of the New York criteria. *Clin Res.* 1983;31:734A.

- van der Linden S, Cats A, Valkenburg HA, Khan MA. Evaluation of the diagnostic criteria for ankylosing spondylitis: a proposal for modification of the New York criteria. *Br J Rheumatol.* 1984;23:148.

- van der Linden SM, Goei The HS, Khan MA, Cats A, Valkenburg HA. Roma locata, causa non finita: parameters that need to be considered in revision of criteria for ankylosing spondylitis and seronegative polyarthritis. *Clin Exp Rheumatol.* 1987;5(Suppl 1):S109–S110.

- van der Linden SM, Khan MA. The risk of ankylosing spondylitis in HLA-B27 positive individuals: a reappraisal [editorial]. *J Rheumatol.* 1984;11:727–728.

- van der Linden SM, Khan MA, Rentsch H-U, et al. Chest pain without radiographic sacroiliitis in relatives of patients with ankylosing spondylitis. *J Rheumatol.* 1988;15:836–839.

- Walsh B, Yocum D, Khan MA. Arthritis and HLA-B27 in North American tribes. *Curr Opin Rheumatol.* 1998;10:319–325.

- Weber U, Pfirrmann CWA, Khan MA. Ankylosing spondylitis: update on imaging and therapy. *Intl J Adv Rheumatol.* 2007;5:2–7.

- Weber U, Pfirrmann CWA, Kissling RO, MacKenzie CR, Khan MA. Early spondyloarthritis in an HLA-B27-positive monozygotic twin pair: a highly concordant onset, sites of involvement, and disease course. *J Rheumatol.* 2008;35(7):1464–1467.

- Whitman GJ, Khan MA. Unusual occurrence of ankylosing spondylitis and multiple sclerosis in a black patient. *Cleve Clin J Med.* 1989;56:819–822.

- Yagan R, Khan MA. Confusion of roentgenographic differential diagnosis between ankylosing hyperostosis (Forestier's disease) and ankylosing spondylitis. *Clin Rheumatol.* 1983;2:285–292.

- Yagan R, Khan MA. Confusion of roentgenographic differential diagnosis of ankylosing hyperostosis (Forestier's disease) and ankylosing spondylitis. *Spine: State of the Art Reviews.* 1990;4:561–575.

- Yagan R, Khan MA, Bellon EM. Spondylitis and posterior longitudinal ligament ossification in the cervical spine. *Arthritis Rheum.* 1983;26:226–230.

- Yagan R, Khan MA, Marmolya G. Role of abdominal CT, when available in patients' records, in the evaluation of degenerative changes of the sacroiliac joints. *Spine.* 1987;12:1046–1051.

- Zanetakis E, Khan MA, Yagan R, Kushner I. Ochronotic arthropathy, spinal pseudoarthrosis and HLA-B27. *J Orthopedic Rheumatol.* 1989;2:48–53.

- Zeidler H, Mau W, Khan MA. Undifferentiated spondyloarthropathies. *Rheum Dis Clin North Am.* 1992;18:187–202.

- Zhang G, Luo J, Bruckel J, et al. Genetic studies in familial ankylosing spondylitis susceptibility. *Arthritis Rheum.* 2004;50:2246–2254.
- Zochling J, van der Heijde D, Burgos-Vargas R, et al. ASAS/EULAR recommendations for the management of ankylosing spondylitis. *Ann Rheum Dis.* 2006;65:442–452.

Index

Page numbers followed by *t* indicate a table; *f* indicates a figure.